# NEURODEVELOPMENTAL
# DISORDERS

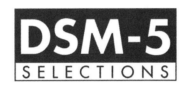

# NEURODEVELOPMENTAL
# DISORDERS

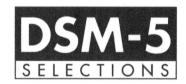

**American Psychiatric Association**

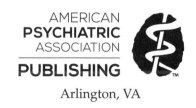

AMERICAN
**PSYCHIATRIC**
ASSOCIATION
**PUBLISHING**

Arlington, VA

Manufactured in the United States of America on acid-free paper.

ISBN 978-1-61537-013-9 (Paperback)

American Psychiatric Association
1000 Wilson Boulevard
Arlington, VA 22209-3901
www.psych.org

*Neurodevelopmental Disorders: DSM-5® Selections* is an anthology published by the American Psychiatric Association from the following sources:

American Psychiatric Association: *Diagnostic and Statistical Manual of Mental Disorders*, Fifth Edition. Arlington, VA, American Psychiatric Association, 2013

Black DW, Grant JE: *DSM-5® Guidebook: The Essential Companion to the Diagnostic and Statistical Manual of Mental Disorders, Fifth Edition*. Washington, DC, American Psychiatric Publishing, 2014

Barnhill JW: *DSM-5® Clinical Cases*. Washington, DC, American Psychiatric Publishing, 2014

Muskin PR: *DSM-5® Self-Exam Questions: Test Questions for the Diagnostic Criteria*. Washington, DC, American Psychiatric Publishing, 2014

# Contents

# Introduction to DSM-5® Selections

Welcome to *DSM-5 Selections*. The purpose of this series is to educate readers about important diagnostic issues associated with categories of DSM-5 disorders. The initial books in the *DSM-5 Selections* series are *Sleep-Wake Disorders, Depressive Disorders, Schizophrenia Spectrum and Other Psychotic Disorders, Feeding and Eating Disorders, Neurodevelopmental Disorders,* and *Anxiety Disorders.* Each book in the series includes the diagnostic criteria relevant to the disorders included in each category. The criteria are taken directly from DSM-5, the most comprehensive, current, and critical resource for clinical practice available today. Also included in each book in the series are extracts from the *DSM-5 Guidebook, DSM-5 Clinical Cases,* and *DSM-5 Self-Exam Questions.* Consequently, each book in the series offers readers a unique introduction to individual categories of DSM-5 disorders and an opportunity to test one's knowledge about DSM-5 disorders.

*DSM-5 Guidebook* serves as a roadmap to DSM-5 disorders for clinicians and researchers. It illuminates the content of DSM-5 by teaching mental health professionals how to use the revised diagnostic criteria, and it provides practical content for its clinical use. The book offers a fresh perspective to DSM diagnostic categories by focusing on the changes between DSM-IV-TR and DSM-5 that will most significantly impact clinical application of the criteria.

*DSM-5 Clinical Cases* presents composite patient cases that exemplify the diagnostic criteria for disorders contained in a category. *DSM-5 Clinical Cases* makes DSM-5 come alive for teachers, students, and clinicians. The book helps readers to understand diagnostic concepts, including symptoms, severity, comorbidities, age of onset and development, dimensionality across disorders, and gender and cultural implications.

The questions in *DSM-5 Self-Exam Questions* were written to test readers' knowledge of conceptual changes to DSM-5, specific changes to diagnoses, and the diagnostic criteria. Each question includes short answers that explain the rationale for each correct answer and contain important information on diagnostic classification, criteria sets, diagnoses, codes, severity, culture, age, and gender. The questions are helpful for preparing for various examinations.

The *DSM-5 Selections* series is not intended to replace DSM-5 or the other books from which the extracts are taken. Rather, the series is intended to give readers key selected materials that pertain directly to specific disorder categories. If you find that you require more information about a specific disorder or category of disorders, you are encouraged to examine an APP textbook or clinical manual. You can review the full list of APP titles at www.appi.org.

Robert E. Hales, M.D.
Editor-in-Chief

# Preface

Included in the diagnostic class of neurodevelopmental disorders are disorders that emerge during childhood or adolescence and that affect behaviors that are important for normal interactions ranging from school to social occasions. Some of the neurodevelopmental disorders, such as intellectual disabilities, will have an effect on multiple domains, and other disorders, such as a specific learning disorder or motor disorder, may be more circumscribed in their effects. A brief summary of some of these disorders is provided here.

*Intellectual disability (intellectual developmental disorder)* is a neurodevelopmental disorder that is characterized by deficits in both intellectual functioning and adaptive functioning relative to peers of the same age and gender and the same linguistic and social cultural background.

The DSM-5 subclass of communication disorders refers to a group of impairments that have an impact on the child's abilities to receive, send, process, and comprehend verbal, nonverbal, and other graphic symbol systems that are shared by a community. *Social (pragmatic) communication disorder* is a new category in DSM-5 and refers to children who have primary difficulty with the pragmatic aspects of language.

*Autism spectrum disorder* now consolidates into one disorder the following disorders that were separate in DSM-TV-TR: autistic disorder, Asperger's disorder, childhood disintegrative disorder, and pervasive developmental disorder not otherwise specified (including atypical autism). Although originally autism was felt to be rare, its estimated prevalence in the United States is now 1 in 88.

*Attention-deficit/hyperactivity disorder* (ADHD) is characterized by developmentally inappropriate persistent problems, inattention, and/or excessive motor restlessness and/or impulsivity that interfere with functioning. It is estimated that between 6% and 7% percent of children have symptoms that meet criteria for ADHD and that approximately 5% of adults may also suffer from this disorder.

A *specific learning disorder* requires persistent difficulties in reading, writing, or arithmetic/mathematical reasoning that emerge during the developmental period and have a significant negative effect on academic performance, occupational functioning, or daily life. *Stereotypic movement disorder* is a condition characterized by repetitive behavior that is driven without purpose and is associated with significant distress and impairment. There are several diagnostic categories of tic disorder; the diagnosis of Tourette's disorder has been estimated to be less than 1%, but diagnosis is higher for chronic tic conditions.

---

Adapted with permission from Abbeduto L, Ozonoff S, Thurman AJ, et al.: "Neurodevelopmental Disorders," in *The American Psychiatric Publishing Textbook of Psychiatry*, 6th Edition. Edited by Hales RE, Yudofsky SC, Roberts LW. Washington, DC, American Psychiatric Publishing, 2014, pp. 229–272.

As can be seen from the brief descriptions of some of the categories of neurodevelopmental disorders, the accurate diagnosis of these conditions requires a systematic and thoughtful evaluation and frequently the use of reliable and valid diagnostic instruments. This selection will provide the details contained within DSM-5 for each of these diagnostic categories. It will also present material to guide identification of the proper disorder and to test the provider's knowledge, and present clinical vignettes that highlight the major characteristics of this constellation of disorders.

# Highlights of Changes From DSM-IV-TR to DSM-5

Changes made to the DSM-5 diagnostic criteria and texts are outlined in this chapter in the same order in which they appear in the DSM-5 classification. This is not an exhaustive guide; minor changes in text or wording made for clarity are not described here. It should also be noted that Section I of DSM-5 contains a description of changes pertaining to the chapter organization in DSM-5, the multiaxial system, and the introduction of dimensional assessments (in Section III).

## Terminology

The phrase *general medical condition* is replaced in DSM-5 with *another medical condition* where relevant across all disorders.

## Intellectual Disability (Intellectual Developmental Disorder)

Diagnostic criteria for intellectual disability (intellectual developmental disorder) emphasize the need for an assessment of both cognitive capacity (IQ) and adaptive functioning. Severity is determined by adaptive functioning rather than IQ score. The term *mental retardation* was used in DSM-IV. However, the term *intellectual disability* has come into common use over the past two decades among medical, educational, and other professionals and by the lay public and advocacy groups. Moreover, a federal statute in the United States (Public Law 111-256, Rosa's Law) replaces the term mental retardation with intellectual disability. Despite the name change, the deficits in cognitive capacity beginning in the developmental period, with the accompanying diagnostic criteria, are considered to constitute a mental disorder. The term intellectual developmental disorder was placed in parentheses to reflect the World Health Organization's classification system, which lists *disorders* in the International Classification of Diseases (ICD; the 11th revision, ICD-11, is expected to be released in 2017) and bases all *disabilities* on the International Classification of Functioning, Disability, and Health (ICF). Because ICD-11 will not be adopted for several years, intellectual disability was chosen as the current preferred term, with the bridge term for the future in parentheses.

## Communication Disorders

The DSM-5 communication disorders include *language disorder* (which combines DSM-IV expressive and mixed receptive-expressive language disorders), *speech sound disorder* (a new name for phonological disorder), and *childhood-onset fluency disorder (stuttering)*. Also included is *social (pragmatic) communication disorder,* a new condition for persistent difficulties in the social uses of verbal and nonverbal communication. Because social communication deficits are one component of *autism spectrum disorder* (ASD), it is important to note that social (pragmatic) communication disorder cannot be diagnosed in the presence of restricted repetitive behaviors, interests, and activities (the other component of ASD). The symptoms of some patients diagnosed with DSM-IV pervasive developmental disorder not otherwise specified may meet the DSM-5 criteria for social (pragmatic) communication disorder.

## Autism Spectrum Disorder

Autism spectrum disorder is a new DSM-5 name that reflects a scientific consensus that four previously separate disorders are actually a single condition with different levels of symptom severity in two core domains. ASD now encompasses the previous DSM-IV autistic disorder, Asperger's disorder, childhood disintegrative disorder, and pervasive developmental disorder not otherwise specified (including atypical autism). ASD is characterized by 1) deficits in social communication and social interaction and 2) restricted repetitive behaviors, interests, and activities (RRBs). Because both components are required for diagnosis of ASD, social (pragmatic) communication disorder is diagnosed if no RRBs are present.

## Attention-Deficit/Hyperactivity Disorder

The diagnostic criteria for ADHD in DSM-5 are similar to those in DSM-IV. The same 18 symptoms are used as in DSM-IV, and they continue to be divided into two symptom domains (inattention and hyperactivity/impulsivity), of which at least 6 symptoms in one domain are required for diagnosis. However, several changes have been made in DSM-5: 1) examples have been added to the criterion items to facilitate application across the life span; 2) the cross-situational requirement has been strengthened to "several" symptoms in each setting; 3) the onset criterion has been changed from "symptoms that caused impairment were present before age 7 years" to "several inattentive or hyperactive-impulsive symptoms were present prior to age 12 years"; 4) subtypes have been replaced with presentation specifiers that map directly to the prior subtypes; 5) a comorbid diagnosis with ASD is now allowed; and 6) a symptom threshold change has been made for adults, to reflect the substantial evidence of clinically significant ADHD impairment, with the cutoff for ADHD of 5 symptoms instead of 6 required for younger persons, both for inattention and for hyperactivity/impulsivity. Finally, ADHD was placed in the "Neurodevelopmental Disorders" chapter to reflect brain developmental correlates with ADHD and the decision in DSM-5 to eliminate the DSM-IV chapter that includes all diagnoses usually first made in infancy, childhood, or adolescence.

## Specific Learning Disorder

Specific learning disorder combines the DSM-IV diagnoses of reading disorder, mathematics disorder, disorder of written expression, and learning disorder not otherwise specified. Because learning deficits in the areas of reading, written expression, and mathematics commonly occur together, coded specifiers for the deficit types in each area are included. The text acknowledges that specific types of reading deficits are described internationally in various ways as dyslexia and specific types of mathematics deficits as dyscalculia.

## Motor Disorders

The following motor disorders are included in the DSM-5 neurodevelopmental disorders chapter: *developmental coordination disorder, stereotypic movement disorder, Tourette's disorder, persistent (chronic) motor or vocal tic disorder, provisional tic disorder, other specified tic disorder,* and *unspecified tic disorder.* The tic criteria have been standardized across all of these disorders in this chapter. Stereotypic movement disorder has been more clearly differentiated from body-focused repetitive behavior disorders, which are discussed in the DSM-5 chapter "Obsessive-Compulsive and Related Disorders."

# DSM-5®
# Neurodevelopmental Disorders: ICD-9-CM and ICD-10-CM Codes

| Disorder | ICD-9-CM | ICD-10-CM |
|---|---|---|
| **Intellectual Disabilities** | | |
| Intellectual Disability (Intellectual Developmental Disorder) | | |
|    Mild | 317 | F70 |
|    Moderate | 318.0 | F71 |
|    Severe | 318.1 | F72 |
|    Profound | 318.2 | F73 |
| Global Developmental Delay | 315.8 | F88 |
| Unspecified Intellectual Disability (Intellectual Developmental Disorder) | 319 | F79 |
| **Communication Disorders** | | |
| Language Disorder | 315.32 | F80.2 |
| Speech Sound Disorder | 315.39 | F80.0 |
| Childhood-Onset Fluency Disorder (Stuttering) | 315.35 | F80.81 |
| Social (Pragmatic) Communication Disorder | 315.39 | F80.89 |
| Unspecified Communication Disorder | 307.9 | F80.9 |
| **Autism Spectrum Disorder** | | |
| Autism Spectrum Disorder | 299.00 | F84.0 |
| **Attention-Deficit/Hyperactivity Disorder** | | |
| Attention-Deficit/Hyperactivity Disorder | | |
|    Combined presentation | 314.01 | F90.2 |
|    Predominantly inattentive presentation | 314.00 | F90.0 |
|    Predominantly hyperactive/impulsive presentation | 314.01 | F90.1 |
| Other Specified Attention-Deficit/Hyperactivity Disorder | 314.01 | F90.8 |
| Unspecified Attention-Deficit/Hyperactivity Disorder | 314.01 | F90.9 |

| Disorder | ICD-9-CM | ICD-10-CM |
|---|---|---|
| **Specific Learning Disorder** | | |
| Specific Learning Disorder | | |
|     With impairment in reading | 315.00 | F81.0 |
|     With impairment in written expression | 315.2 | F81.81 |
|     With impairment in mathematics | 315.1 | F81.2 |
| **Motor Disorders** | | |
| Developmental Coordination Disorder | 315.4 | F82 |
| Stereotypic Movement Disorder | 307.3 | F98.4 |
| Tic Disorders | | |
|     Tourette's Disorder | 307.23 | F95.2 |
|     Persistent (Chronic) Motor or Vocal Tic Disorder | 307.22 | F95.1 |
|     Provisional Tic Disorder | 307.21 | F95.0 |
|     Other Specified Tic Disorder | 307.20 | F95.8 |
|     Unspecified Tic Disorder | 307.20 | F95.9 |
| **Other Neurodevelopmental Disorders** | | |
| Other Specified Neurodevelopmental Disorder | 315.8 | F88 |
| Unspecified Neurodevelopmental Disorder | 315.9 | F89 |

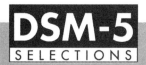

# Neurodevelopmental Disorders

## Diagnostic and Statistical Manual of Mental Disorders, Fifth Edition

The neurodevelopmental disorders are a group of conditions with onset in the developmental period. The disorders typically manifest early in development, often before the child enters grade school, and are characterized by developmental deficits that produce impairments of personal, social, academic, or occupational functioning. The range of developmental deficits varies from very specific limitations of learning or control of executive functions to global impairments of social skills or intelligence. The neurodevelopmental disorders frequently co-occur; for example, individuals with autism spectrum disorder often have intellectual disability (intellectual developmental disorder), and many children with attention-deficit/hyperactivity disorder (ADHD) also have a specific learning disorder. For some disorders, the clinical presentation includes symptoms of excess as well as deficits and delays in achieving expected milestones. For example, autism spectrum disorder is diagnosed only when the characteristic deficits of social communication are accompanied by excessively repetitive behaviors, restricted interests, and insistence on sameness.

Intellectual disability (intellectual developmental disorder) is characterized by deficits in general mental abilities, such as reasoning, problem solving, planning, abstract thinking, judgment, academic learning, and learning from experience. The deficits result in impairments of adaptive functioning, such that the individual fails to meet standards of personal independence and social responsibility in one or more aspects of daily life, including communication, social participation, academic or occupational functioning, and personal independence at home or in community settings. Global developmental delay, as its name implies, is diagnosed when an individual fails to meet expected developmental milestones in several areas of intellectual functioning. The diagnosis is used for individuals who are unable to undergo systematic assessments of intellectual functioning, including children who are too young to participate in standardized testing. Intellectual disability may result from an acquired insult during the developmental period from, for example, a severe head injury, in which case a neurocognitive disorder also may be diagnosed.

The communication disorders include language disorder, speech sound disorder, social (pragmatic) communication disorder, and childhood-onset fluency disorder (stuttering). The first three disorders are characterized by deficits in the development and use of language, speech, and social communication, respectively. Childhood-onset fluency disorder is characterized by disturbances of the normal fluency and motor production of speech, including repetitive sounds or syllables, prolongation of consonants or vowel sounds, broken words, blocking, or words produced with an excess of physical tension. Like other neurodevelopmental disorders, communication disorders begin early in life and may produce lifelong functional impairments.

Autism spectrum disorder is characterized by persistent deficits in social communication and social interaction across multiple contexts, including deficits in social reciprocity, nonverbal communicative behaviors used for social interaction, and skills in developing, maintaining, and understanding relationships. In addition to the social communication deficits, the diagnosis of autism spectrum disorder requires the presence of restricted, repetitive patterns of behavior, interests, or activities. Because symptoms change with development and may be masked by compensatory mechanisms, the diagnostic criteria may be met based on historical information, although the current presentation must cause significant impairment.

Within the diagnosis of autism spectrum disorder, individual clinical characteristics are noted through the use of specifiers (with or without accompanying intellectual impairment; with or without accompanying structural language impairment; associated with a known medical or genetic condition or environmental factor; associated with another neurodevelopmental, mental, or behavioral disorder), as well as specifiers that describe the autistic symptoms (age at first concern; with or without loss of established skills; severity). These specifiers provide clinicians with an opportunity to individualize the diagnosis and communicate a richer clinical description of the affected individuals. For example, many individuals previously diagnosed with Asperger's disorder would now receive a diagnosis of autism spectrum disorder without language or intellectual impairment.

ADHD is a neurodevelopmental disorder defined by impairing levels of inattention, disorganization, and/or hyperactivity-impulsivity. Inattention and disorganization entail inability to stay on task, seeming not to listen, and losing materials, at levels that are inconsistent with age or developmental level. Hyperactivity-impulsivity entails overactivity, fidgeting, inability to stay seated, intruding into other people's activities, and inability to wait—symptoms that are excessive for age or developmental level. In childhood, ADHD frequently overlaps with disorders that are often considered to be "externalizing disorders," such as oppositional defiant disorder and conduct disorder. ADHD often persists into adulthood, with resultant impairments of social, academic and occupational functioning.

The neurodevelopmental motor disorders include developmental coordination disorder, stereotypic movement disorder, and tic disorders. Developmental coordination disorder is characterized by deficits in the acquisition and execution of coordinated motor skills and is manifested by clumsiness and slowness or inaccuracy of performance of motor skills that cause interference with activities of daily living. Stereotypic movement disorder is diagnosed when an individual has repetitive, seemingly driven, and apparently purposeless motor behaviors, such as hand flapping, body rocking, head banging, self-biting, or hitting. The movements interfere with social, academic, or other activities. If the behaviors cause self-injury, this should be specified as part of the diagnostic description. Tic disorders are characterized by the presence of motor or vocal tics, which are sudden, rapid, recurrent, nonrhythmic, stereotyped motor movements or vocalizations. The duration, presumed etiology, and clinical presentation define the specific tic disorder that is diagnosed: Tourette's disorder, persistent (chronic) motor or vocal tic disorder, provisional tic disorder, other specified tic disorder, and unspecified tic disorder. Tourette's disorder is diagnosed when the individual has multiple motor and vocal tics that have been present for at least 1 year and that have a waxing-waning symptom course.

Specific learning disorder, as the name implies, is diagnosed when there are specific deficits in an individual's ability to perceive or process information efficiently and accurately. This neurodevelopmental disorder first manifests during the years of formal schooling and is characterized by persistent and impairing difficulties with learning foundational academic skills in reading, writing, and/or math. The individual's performance of the affected academic skills is well below average for age, or acceptable performance levels are achieved only with extraordinary effort. Specific learning disorder may occur in individuals identified as intellectually gifted and manifest only when the learning demands or assessment procedures (e.g., timed tests) pose barriers that cannot be overcome by their innate intelligence and compensatory strategies. For all individuals, specific learning disorder can produce lifelong impairments in activities dependent on the skills, including occupational performance.

The use of specifiers for the neurodevelopmental disorder diagnoses enriches the clinical description of the individual's clinical course and current symptomatology. In addition to specifiers that describe the clinical presentation, such as age at onset or severity ratings, the neurodevelopmental disorders may include the specifier "associated with a known medical or genetic condition or environmental factor." This specifier gives clinicians an opportunity to document factors that may have played a role in the etiology of the disorder, as well as those that might affect the clinical course. Examples include genetic disorders, such as fragile X syndrome, tuberous sclerosis, and Rett syndrome; medical conditions such as epilepsy; and environmental factors, including very low birth weight and fetal alcohol exposure (even in the absence of stigmata of fetal alcohol syndrome).

# Intellectual Disabilities

## Intellectual Disability (Intellectual Developmental Disorder)

### Diagnostic Criteria

Intellectual disability (intellectual developmental disorder) is a disorder with onset during the developmental period that includes both intellectual and adaptive functioning deficits in conceptual, social, and practical domains. The following three criteria must be met:

A. Deficits in intellectual functions, such as reasoning, problem solving, planning, abstract thinking, judgment, academic learning, and learning from experience, confirmed by both clinical assessment and individualized, standardized intelligence testing.

B. Deficits in adaptive functioning that result in failure to meet developmental and sociocultural standards for personal independence and social responsibility. Without ongoing support, the adaptive deficits limit functioning in one or more activities of daily life, such as communication, social participation, and independent living, across multiple environments, such as home, school, work, and community.

C. Onset of intellectual and adaptive deficits during the developmental period.

**Note:** The diagnostic term *intellectual disability* is the equivalent term for the ICD-11 diagnosis of *intellectual developmental disorders.* Although the term *intellectual disability* is used throughout this manual, both terms are used in the title to clarify relationships with other classification systems. Moreover, a federal statute in the United States (Public Law 111-256, Rosa's Law) replaces the term *mental retardation* with *intellectual disability,* and research journals use the term *intellectual disability.* Thus, *intellectual disability* is the term in common use by medical, educational, and other professions and by the lay public and advocacy groups.

*Specify* current severity (see Table 1 [pp. 5–7 below; DSM-5, pp. 34–36]):

**317 (F70)   Mild**
**318.0 (F71) Moderate**
**318.1 (F72) Severe**
**318.2 (F73) Profound**

## Specifiers

The various levels of severity are defined on the basis of adaptive functioning, and not IQ scores, because it is adaptive functioning that determines the level of supports required. Moreover, IQ measures are less valid in the lower end of the IQ range.

## Diagnostic Features

The essential features of intellectual disability (intellectual developmental disorder) are deficits in general mental abilities (Criterion A) and impairment in everyday adaptive functioning, in comparison to an individual's age-, gender-, and socioculturally matched peers (Criterion B). Onset is during the developmental period (Criterion C). The diagnosis of intellectual disability is based on both clinical assessment and standardized testing of intellectual and adaptive functions.

Criterion A refers to intellectual functions that involve reasoning, problem solving, planning, abstract thinking, judgment, learning from instruction and experience, and practical understanding. Critical components include verbal comprehension, working memory, perceptual reasoning, quantitative reasoning, abstract thought, and cognitive efficacy. Intellectual functioning is typically measured with individually administered and psychometrically valid, comprehensive, culturally appropriate, psychometrically sound tests of intelligence. Individuals with intellectual disability have scores of approximately two standard deviations or more below the population mean, including a margin for measurement error (generally +5 points). On tests with a standard deviation of 15 and a mean of 100, this involves a score of 65–75 ($70 \pm 5$). Clinical training and judgment are required to interpret test results and assess intellectual performance.

**TABLE 1    Severity levels for intellectual disability (intellectual developmental disorder)**

| Severity level | Conceptual domain | Social domain | Practical domain |
|---|---|---|---|
| Mild | For preschool children, there may be no obvious conceptual differences. For school-age children and adults, there are difficulties in learning academic skills involving reading, writing, arithmetic, time, or money, with support needed in one or more areas to meet age-related expectations. In adults, abstract thinking, executive function (i.e., planning, strategizing, priority setting, and cognitive flexibility), and short-term memory, as well as functional use of academic skills (e.g., reading, money management), are impaired. There is a somewhat concrete approach to problems and solutions compared with age-mates. | Compared with typically developing age-mates, the individual is immature in social interactions. For example, there may be difficulty in accurately perceiving peers' social cues. Communication, conversation, and language are more concrete or immature than expected for age. There may be difficulties regulating emotion and behavior in age-appropriate fashion; these difficulties are noticed by peers in social situations. There is limited understanding of risk in social situations; social judgment is immature for age, and the person is at risk of being manipulated by others (gullibility). | The individual may function age-appropriately in personal care. Individuals need some support with complex daily living tasks in comparison to peers. In adulthood, supports typically involve grocery shopping, transportation, home and child-care organizing, nutritious food preparation, and banking and money management. Recreational skills resemble those of age-mates, although judgment related to well-being and organization around recreation requires support. In adulthood, competitive employment is often seen in jobs that do not emphasize conceptual skills. Individuals generally need support to make health care decisions and legal decisions, and to learn to perform a skilled vocation competently. Support is typically needed to raise a family. |

**TABLE 1   Severity levels for intellectual disability (intellectual developmental disorder)** *(continued)*

| Severity level | Conceptual domain | Social domain | Practical domain |
|---|---|---|---|
| Moderate | All through development, the individual's conceptual skills lag markedly behind those of peers. For preschoolers, language and pre-academic skills develop slowly. For school-age children, progress in reading, writing, mathematics, and understanding of time and money occurs slowly across the school years and is markedly limited compared with that of peers. For adults, academic skill development is typically at an elementary level, and support is required for all use of academic skills in work and personal life. Ongoing assistance on a daily basis is needed to complete conceptual tasks of day-to-day life, and others may take over these responsibilities fully for the individual. | The individual shows marked differences from peers in social and communicative behavior across development. Spoken language is typically a primary tool for social communication but is much less complex than that of peers. Capacity for relationships is evident in ties to family and friends, and the individual may have successful friendships across life and sometimes romantic relations in adulthood. However, individuals may not perceive or interpret social cues accurately. Social judgment and decision-making abilities are limited, and caretakers must assist the person with life decisions. Friendships with typically developing peers are often affected by communication or social limitations. Significant social and communicative support is needed in work settings for success. | The individual can care for personal needs involving eating, dressing, elimination, and hygiene as an adult, although an extended period of teaching and time is needed for the individual to become independent in these areas, and reminders may be needed. Similarly, participation in all household tasks can be achieved by adulthood, although an extended period of teaching is needed, and ongoing supports will typically occur for adult-level performance. Independent employment in jobs that require limited conceptual and communication skills can be achieved, but considerable support from co-workers, supervisors, and others is needed to manage social expectations, job complexities, and ancillary responsibilities such as scheduling, transportation, health benefits, and money management. A variety of recreational skills can be developed. These typically require additional supports and learning opportunities over an extended period of time. Maladaptive behavior is present in a significant minority and causes social problems. |

**TABLE 1** Severity levels for intellectual disability (intellectual developmental disorder) (*continued*)

| Severity level | Conceptual domain | Social domain | Practical domain |
|---|---|---|---|
| Severe | Attainment of conceptual skills is limited. The individual generally has little understanding of written language or of concepts involving numbers, quantity, time, and money. Caretakers provide extensive supports for problem solving throughout life. | Spoken language is quite limited in terms of vocabulary and grammar. Speech may be single words or phrases and may be supplemented through augmentative means. Speech and communication are focused on the here and now within everyday events. Language is used for social communication more than for explication. Individuals understand simple speech and gestural communication. Relationships with family members and familiar others are a source of pleasure and help. | The individual requires support for all activities of daily living, including meals, dressing, bathing, and elimination. The individual requires supervision at all times. The individual cannot make responsible decisions regarding well-being of self or others. In adulthood, participation in tasks at home, recreation, and work requires ongoing support and assistance. Skill acquisition in all domains involves long-term teaching and ongoing support. Maladaptive behavior, including self-injury, is present in a significant minority. |
| Profound | Conceptual skills generally involve the physical world rather than symbolic processes. The individual may use objects in goal-directed fashion for self-care, work, and recreation. Certain visuospatial skills, such as matching and sorting based on physical characteristics, may be acquired. However, co-occurring motor and sensory impairments may prevent functional use of objects. | The individual has very limited understanding of symbolic communication in speech or gesture. He or she may understand some simple instructions or gestures. The individual expresses his or her own desires and emotions largely through nonverbal, nonsymbolic communication. The individual enjoys relationships with well-known family members, caretakers, and familiar others, and initiates and responds to social interactions through gestural and emotional cues. Co-occurring sensory and physical impairments may prevent many social activities. | The individual is dependent on others for all aspects of daily physical care, health, and safety, although he or she may be able to participate in some of these activities as well. Individuals without severe physical impairments may assist with some daily work tasks at home, like carrying dishes to the table. Simple actions with objects may be the basis of participation in some vocational activities with high levels of ongoing support. Recreational activities may involve, for example, enjoyment in listening to music, watching movies, going out for walks, or participating in water activities, all with the support of others. Co-occurring physical and sensory impairments are frequent barriers to participation (beyond watching) in home, recreational, and vocational activities. Maladaptive behavior is present in a significant minority. |

Factors that may affect test scores include practice effects and the "Flynn effect" (i.e., overly high scores due to out-of-date test norms). Invalid scores may result from the use of brief intelligence screening tests or group tests; highly discrepant individual subtest scores may make an overall IQ score invalid. Instruments must be normed for the individual's sociocultural background and native language. Co-occurring disorders that affect communication, language, and/or motor or sensory function may affect test scores. Individual cognitive profiles based on neuropsychological testing are more useful for understanding intellectual abilities than a single IQ score. Such testing may identify areas of relative strengths and weaknesses, an assessment important for academic and vocational planning.

IQ test scores are approximations of conceptual functioning but may be insufficient to assess reasoning in real-life situations and mastery of practical tasks. For example, a person with an IQ score above 70 may have such severe adaptive behavior problems in social judgment, social understanding, and other areas of adaptive functioning that the person's actual functioning is comparable to that of individuals with a lower IQ score. Thus, clinical judgment is needed in interpreting the results of IQ tests.

Deficits in adaptive functioning (Criterion B) refer to how well a person meets community standards of personal independence and social responsibility, in comparison to others of similar age and sociocultural background. Adaptive functioning involves adaptive reasoning in three domains: conceptual, social, and practical. The *conceptual (academic) domain* involves competence in memory, language, reading, writing, math reasoning, acquisition of practical knowledge, problem solving, and judgment in novel situations, among others. The *social domain* involves awareness of others' thoughts, feelings, and experiences; empathy; interpersonal communication skills; friendship abilities; and social judgment, among others. The *practical domain* involves learning and self-management across life settings, including personal care, job responsibilities, money management, recreation, self-management of behavior, and school and work task organization, among others. Intellectual capacity, education, motivation, socialization, personality features, vocational opportunity, cultural experience, and coexisting general medical conditions or mental disorders influence adaptive functioning.

Adaptive functioning is assessed using both clinical evaluation and individualized, culturally appropriate, psychometrically sound measures. Standardized measures are used with knowledgeable informants (e.g., parent or other family member; teacher; counselor; care provider) and the individual to the extent possible. Additional sources of information include educational, developmental, medical, and mental health evaluations. Scores from standardized measures and interview sources must be interpreted using clinical judgment. When standardized testing is difficult or impossible, because of a variety of factors (e.g., sensory impairment, severe problem behavior), the individual may be diagnosed with unspecified intellectual disability. Adaptive functioning may be difficult to assess in a controlled setting (e.g., prisons, detention centers); if possible, corroborative information reflecting functioning outside those settings should be obtained.

Criterion B is met when at least one domain of adaptive functioning—conceptual, social, or practical—is sufficiently impaired that ongoing support is needed in order for the person to perform adequately in one or more life settings at school, at work, at home, or in the community. To meet diagnostic criteria for intellectual disability, the deficits in adaptive functioning must be directly related to the intellectual impairments described in Criterion A. Criterion C, onset during the developmental period, refers to recognition that intellectual and adaptive deficits are present during childhood or adolescence.

## Associated Features Supporting Diagnosis

Intellectual disability is a heterogeneous condition with multiple causes. There may be associated difficulties with social judgment; assessment of risk; self-management of behavior, emotions, or interpersonal relationships; or motivation in school or work environments. Lack of communication skills may predispose to disruptive and aggressive behaviors. Gullibility is often a feature, involving naiveté in social situations and a tendency for being easily led by others. Gullibility and lack of awareness of risk may result in exploitation by others and possible victimization, fraud, unintentional criminal involvement, false confessions, and risk for physical and sexual abuse. These associated features can be important in criminal cases, including Atkins-type hearings involving the death penalty.

Individuals with a diagnosis of intellectual disability with co-occurring mental disorders are at risk for suicide. They think about suicide, make suicide attempts, and may die from them. Thus, screening for suicidal thoughts is essential in the assessment process. Because of a lack of awareness of risk and danger, accidental injury rates may be increased.

## Prevalence

Intellectual disability has an overall general population prevalence of approximately 1%, and prevalence rates vary by age. Prevalence for severe intellectual disability is approximately 6 per 1,000.

## Development and Course

Onset of intellectual disability is in the developmental period. The age and characteristic features at onset depend on the etiology and severity of brain dysfunction. Delayed motor, language, and social milestones may be identifiable within the first 2 years of life among those with more severe intellectual disability, while mild levels may not be identifiable until school age when difficulty with academic learning becomes apparent. All criteria (including Criterion C) must be fulfilled by history or current presentation. Some children under age 5 years whose presentation will eventually meet criteria for intellectual disability have deficits that meet criteria for global developmental delay.

When intellectual disability is associated with a genetic syndrome, there may be a characteristic physical appearance (as in, e.g., Down syndrome). Some syndromes have a *behavioral phenotype,* which refers to specific behaviors that are characteristic of particular genetic disorder (e.g., Lesch-Nyhan syndrome). In acquired forms, the onset may be abrupt following an illness such as meningitis or encephalitis or head trauma occurring during the developmental period. When intellectual disability results from a loss of previously acquired cognitive skills, as in severe traumatic brain injury, the diagnoses of intellectual disability and of a neurocognitive disorder may both be assigned.

Although intellectual disability is generally nonprogressive, in certain genetic disorders (e.g., Rett syndrome) there are periods of worsening, followed by stabilization, and in others (e.g., San Phillippo syndrome) progressive worsening of intellectual function. After early childhood, the disorder is generally lifelong, although severity levels may change over time. The course may be influenced by underlying medical or genetic conditions and co-occurring conditions (e.g., hearing or visual impairments, epilepsy). Early and ongoing interventions may improve adaptive functioning throughout childhood and adulthood. In some cases, these result in significant improvement of intellectual functioning, such that the diagnosis of intellectual disability is no longer appropriate. Thus, it is common practice when assessing infants and young children to delay diagnosis of intellectual disability until after an appropriate course of intervention is provided. For older children and adults, the extent of support provided may allow for full participation in all activities of daily living and improved adaptive function. Diagnostic assessments must determine whether improved adaptive skills are the result of a stable, generalized new skill acquisition (in which case the diagnosis of intellectual disability may no longer be appropriate) or whether the improvement is contingent on the presence of supports and ongoing interventions (in which case the diagnosis of intellectual disability may still be appropriate).

## Risk and Prognostic Factors

**Genetic and physiological.**   Prenatal etiologies include genetic syndromes (e.g., sequence variations or copy number variants involving one or more genes; chromosomal disorders), inborn errors of metabolism, brain malformations, maternal disease (including placental disease), and environmental influences (e.g., alcohol, other drugs, toxins, teratogens). Perinatal causes include a variety of labor and delivery-related events leading to neonatal encephalopathy. Postnatal causes include hypoxic ischemic injury, traumatic brain injury, infections, demyelinating disorders, seizure disorders (e.g., infantile spasms), severe and chronic social deprivation, and toxic metabolic syndromes and intoxications (e.g., lead, mercury).

## Culture-Related Diagnostic Issues

Intellectual disability occurs in all races and cultures. Cultural sensitivity and knowledge are needed during assessment, and the individual's ethnic, cultural, and linguistic background, available experiences, and adaptive functioning within his or her community and cultural setting must be taken into account.

## Gender-Related Diagnostic Issues

Overall, males are more likely than females to be diagnosed with both mild (average male:female ratio 1.6:1) and severe (average male:female ratio 1.2:1) forms of intellectual disability. However, gender ratios vary widely in reported studies. Sex-linked genetic factors and male vulnerability to brain insult may account for some of the gender differences.

## Diagnostic Markers

A comprehensive evaluation includes an assessment of intellectual capacity and adaptive functioning; identification of genetic and nongenetic etiologies; evaluation for associated medical conditions (e.g., cerebral palsy, seizure disorder); and evaluation for co-occurring mental, emotional, and behavioral disorders. Components of the evaluation may include basic pre- and perinatal medical history, three-generational family pedigree, physical examination, genetic evaluation (e.g., karyotype or chromosomal microarray analysis and testing for specific genetic syndromes), and metabolic screening and neuroimaging assessment.

## Differential Diagnosis

The diagnosis of intellectual disability should be made whenever Criteria A, B, and C are met. A diagnosis of intellectual disability should not be assumed because of a particular genetic or medical condition. A genetic syndrome linked to intellectual disability should be noted as a concurrent diagnosis with the intellectual disability.

**Major and mild neurocognitive disorders.**   Intellectual disability is categorized as a neurodevelopmental disorder and is distinct from the neurocognitive disorders, which are characterized by a loss of cognitive functioning. Major neurocognitive disorder may co-occur with intellectual disability (e.g., an individual with Down syndrome who develops Alzheimer's disease, or an individual with intellectual disability who loses further cognitive capacity following a head injury). In such cases, the diagnoses of intellectual disability and neurocognitive disorder may both be given.

**Communication disorders and specific learning disorder.**   These neurodevelopmental disorders are specific to the communication and learning domains and do not show deficits in intellectual and adaptive behavior. They may co-occur with intellectual disability. Both diagnoses are made if full criteria are met for intellectual disability and a communication disorder or specific learning disorder.

**Autism spectrum disorder.**   Intellectual disability is common among individuals with autism spectrum disorder. Assessment of intellectual ability may be complicated by social-communication and behavior deficits inherent to autism spectrum disorder, which may interfere with understanding and complying with test procedures. Appropriate assessment of intellectual functioning in autism spectrum disorder is essential, with reassessment across the developmental period, because IQ scores in autism spectrum disorder may be unstable, particularly in early childhood.

## Comorbidity

Co-occurring mental, neurodevelopmental, medical, and physical conditions are frequent in intellectual disability, with rates of some conditions (e.g., mental disorders, cerebral palsy, and epilepsy) three to four times higher than in the general population. The prognosis and outcome of co-occurring diagnoses may be influenced by the presence of intellectual disability. Assessment procedures may require modifications because of associated disorders, including communication disorders, autism spectrum disorder, and motor, sensory, or other disorders. Knowledgeable informants are essential for identifying symptoms such as irritability, mood dysregulation, aggression, eating problems, and sleep problems, and for assessing adaptive functioning in various community settings.

The most common co-occurring mental and neurodevelopmental disorders are attention-deficit/hyperactivity disorder; depressive and bipolar disorders; anxiety disorders; autism spectrum disorder; stereotypic movement disorder (with or without self-injurious behavior); impulse-control disorders; and major neurocognitive disorder. Major depressive disorder may occur throughout the range of severity of intellectual disability. Self-injurious behavior requires prompt diagnostic attention and may warrant a separate diagnosis of stereotypic movement disorder. Individuals with intellectual disability, particularly those with more severe intellectual disability, may also exhibit aggression and disruptive behaviors, including harm of others or property destruction.

## Relationship to Other Classifications

ICD-11 (in development at the time of this publication) uses the term *intellectual developmental disorders* to indicate that these are disorders that involve impaired brain functioning early in life. These disorders are described in ICD-11 as a metasyndrome occurring in the developmental period analogous to dementia or neurocognitive disorder in later life. There are four subtypes in ICD-11: mild, moderate, severe, and profound.

The American Association on Intellectual and Developmental Disabilities (AAIDD) also uses the term *intellectual disability* with a similar meaning to the term as used in this manual. The AAIDD's classification is multidimensional rather than categorical and is based on the disability construct. Rather than listing specifiers as is done in DSM-5, the AAIDD emphasizes a profile of supports based on severity.

# Global Developmental Delay

## 315.8 (F88)

This diagnosis is reserved for individuals *under* the age of 5 years when the clinical severity level cannot be reliably assessed during early childhood. This category is diagnosed when an individual fails to meet expected developmental milestones in several areas of intellectual functioning, and applies to individuals who are unable to undergo systematic assessments of intellectual functioning, including children who are too young to participate in standardized testing. This category requires reassessment after a period of time.

# Unspecified Intellectual Disability (Intellectual Developmental Disorder)

## 319 (F79)

This category is reserved for individuals *over* the age of 5 years when assessment of the degree of intellectual disability (intellectual developmental disorder) by means of locally available procedures is rendered difficult or impossible because of associated sensory or physical impairments, as in blindness or prelingual deafness; locomotor disability; or presence of severe problem behaviors or co-occurring mental disorder. This category should only be used in exceptional circumstances and requires reassessment after a period of time.

# Communication Disorders

Disorders of communication include deficits in language, speech, and communication. *Speech* is the expressive production of sounds and includes an individual's articulation, fluency, voice, and resonance quality. *Language* includes the form, function, and use of a conventional system of symbols (i.e., spoken words, sign language, written words, pictures) in a rule-governed manner for communication. *Communication* includes any verbal or nonverbal behavior (whether intentional or unintentional) that influences the behavior, ideas, or attitudes of another individual. Assessments of speech, language and communication abilities must take into account the individual's cultural and language context, particularly for individuals growing up in bilingual environments. The standardized measures of language development and of nonverbal intellectual capacity must be relevant for the cultural and linguistic group (i.e., tests developed and standardized for one group may not provide appropriate norms for a different group). The diagnostic category of communication disorders includes the following: language disorder, speech sound disorder, childhood-onset fluency disorder (stuttering), social (pragmatic) communication disorder, and other specified and unspecified communication disorders.

## Language Disorder

Diagnostic Criteria                                      **315.32 (F80.2)**

A. Persistent difficulties in the acquisition and use of language across modalities (i.e., spoken, written, sign language, or other) due to deficits in comprehension or production that include the following:

1. Reduced vocabulary (word knowledge and use).
2. Limited sentence structure (ability to put words and word endings together to form sentences based on the rules of grammar and morphology).
3. Impairments in discourse (ability to use vocabulary and connect sentences to explain or describe a topic or series of events or have a conversation).

B. Language abilities are substantially and quantifiably below those expected for age, resulting in functional limitations in effective communication, social participation, academic achievement, or occupational performance, individually or in any combination.

C. Onset of symptoms is in the early developmental period.

D. The difficulties are not attributable to hearing or other sensory impairment, motor dysfunction, or another medical or neurological condition and are not better explained by intellectual disability (intellectual developmental disorder) or global developmental delay.

## Diagnostic Features

The core diagnostic features of language disorder are difficulties in the acquisition and use of language due to deficits in the comprehension or production of vocabulary, sentence structure, and discourse. The language deficits are evident in spoken communication, written communication, or sign language. Language learning and use is dependent on both receptive and expressive skills. *Expressive ability* refers to the production of vocal, gestural, or verbal signals, while *receptive ability* refers to the process of receiving and comprehending language messages. Language skills need to be assessed in both expressive and receptive modalities as these may differ in severity. For example, an individual's expressive language may be severely impaired, while his receptive language is hardly impaired at all.

Language disorder usually affects vocabulary and grammar, and these effects then limit the capacity for discourse. The child's first words and phrases are likely to be delayed in onset; vocabulary size is smaller and less varied than expected; and sentences are shorter and less complex with grammatical errors, especially in past tense. Deficits in comprehension of language are frequently underestimated, as children may be good at using context to infer meaning. There may be word-finding problems, impoverished verbal definitions, or poor understanding of synonyms, multiple meanings, or word play appropriate for age and culture. Problems with remembering new words and sentences are manifested by difficulties following instructions of increasing length, difficulties rehearsing strings of verbal information (e.g., remembering a phone number or a shopping list), and difficulties remembering novel sound sequences, a skill that may be important for learning new words. Difficulties with discourse are shown by a reduced ability to provide adequate information about the key events and to narrate a coherent story.

The language difficulty is manifest by abilities substantially and quantifiably below that expected for age and significantly interfering with academic achievement, occupational performance, effective communication, or socialization (Criterion B). A diagnosis of language disorder is made based on the synthesis of the individual's history, direct clinical observation in different contexts (i.e., home, school, or work), and scores from standardized tests of language ability that can be used to guide estimates of severity.

## Associated Features Supporting Diagnosis

A positive family history of language disorders is often present. Individuals, even children, can be adept at accommodating to their limited language. They may appear to be shy or reticent to talk. Affected individuals may prefer to communicate only with family members or other familiar individuals. Although these social indicators are not diagnostic of a language disorder, if they are notable and persistent, they warrant referral for a full language assessment. Language disorder, particularly expressive deficits, may co-occur with speech sound disorder.

## Development and Course

Language acquisition is marked by changes from onset in toddlerhood to the adult level of competency that appears during adolescence. Changes appear across the dimensions of language (sounds, words, grammar, narratives/expository texts, and conversational skills) in age-graded increments and synchronies. Language disorder emerges during the early developmental period; however, there is considerable variation in early vocabulary acquisition and early word combinations, and individual differences are not, as single indicators, highly predictive of later outcomes. By age 4 years, individual differences in language ability are more stable, with better measurement accuracy, and are highly predictive of later outcomes. Language disorder diagnosed from 4 years of age is likely to be stable over time and typically persists into adulthood, although the particular profile of language strengths and deficits is likely to change over the course of development.

## Risk and Prognostic Factors

Children with receptive language impairments have a poorer prognosis than those with predominantly expressive impairments. They are more resistant to treatment, and difficulties with reading comprehension are frequently seen.

**Genetic and physiological.** Language disorders are highly heritable, and family members are more likely to have a history of language impairment.

## Differential Diagnosis

**Normal variations in language.** Language disorder needs to be distinguished from normal developmental variations, and this distinction may be difficult to make before 4 years of age. Regional, social, or cultural/ethnic variations of language (e.g., dialects) must be considered when an individual is being assessed for language impairment.

**Hearing or other sensory impairment.** Hearing impairment needs to be excluded as the primary cause of language difficulties. Language deficits may be associated with a hearing impairment, other sensory deficit, or a speech-motor deficit. When language deficits are in excess of those usually associated with these problems, a diagnosis of language disorder may be made.

**Intellectual disability (intellectual developmental disorder).** Language delay is often the presenting feature of intellectual disability, and the definitive diagnosis may not be made until the child is able to complete standardized assessments. A separate diagnosis is not given unless the language deficits are clearly in excess of the intellectual limitations.

**Neurological disorders.** Language disorder can be acquired in association with neurological disorders, including epilepsy (e.g., acquired aphasia or Landau-Kleffner syndrome).

**Language regression.**   Loss of speech and language in a child younger than 3 years may be a sign of autism spectrum disorder (with developmental regression) or a specific neurological condition, such as Landau-Kleffner syndrome. Among children older than 3 years, language loss may be a symptom of seizures, and a diagnostic assessment is necessary to exclude the presence of epilepsy (e.g., routine and sleep electroencephalogram).

## Comorbidity

Language disorder is strongly associated with other neurodevelopmental disorders in terms of specific learning disorder (literacy and numeracy), attention-deficit/hyperactivity disorder, autism spectrum disorder, and developmental coordination disorder. It is also associated with social (pragmatic) communication disorder. A positive family history of speech or language disorders is often present.

# Speech Sound Disorder

Diagnostic Criteria                                                           **315.39** (F80.0)

A. Persistent difficulty with speech sound production that interferes with speech intelligibility or prevents verbal communication of messages.
B. The disturbance causes limitations in effective communication that interfere with social participation, academic achievement, or occupational performance, individually or in any combination.
C. Onset of symptoms is in the early developmental period.
D. The difficulties are not attributable to congenital or acquired conditions, such as cerebral palsy, cleft palate, deafness or hearing loss, traumatic brain injury, or other medical or neurological conditions.

## Diagnostic Features

Speech sound production describes the clear articulation of the phonemes (i.e., individual sounds) that in combination make up spoken words. Speech sound production requires both the phonological knowledge of speech sounds and the ability to coordinate the movements of the articulators (i.e., the jaw, tongue, and lips,) with breathing and vocalizing for speech. Children with speech production difficulties may experience difficulty with phonological knowledge of speech sounds or the ability to coordinate movements for speech in varying degrees. Speech sound disorder is thus heterogeneous in its underlying mechanisms and includes phonological disorder and articulation disorder. A speech sound disorder is diagnosed when speech sound production is not what would be expected based on the child's age and developmental stage and when the deficits are not the result of a physical, structural, neurological, or hearing impairment. Among typically developing children at age 4 years, overall speech should be intelligible, whereas at age 2 years, only 50% may be understandable.

# Associated Features Supporting Diagnosis

Language disorder, particularly expressive deficits, may be found to co-occur with speech sound disorder. A positive family history of speech or language disorders is often present.

If the ability to rapidly coordinate the articulators is a particular aspect of difficulty, there may be a history of delay or incoordination in acquiring skills that also utilize the articulators and related facial musculature; among others, these skills include chewing, maintaining mouth closure, and blowing the nose. Other areas of motor coordination may be impaired as in developmental coordination disorder. *Verbal dyspraxia* is a term also used for speech production problems.

Speech may be differentially impaired in certain genetic conditions (e.g., Down syndrome, 22q deletion, *FoxP2* gene mutation). If present, these should also be coded.

# Development and Course

Learning to produce speech sounds clearly and accurately and learning to produce connected speech fluently are developmental skills. Articulation of speech sounds follows a developmental pattern, which is reflected in the age norms of standardized tests. It is not unusual for typically developing children to use developmental processes for shortening words and syllables as they are learning to talk, but their progression in mastering speech sound production should result in mostly intelligible speech by age 3 years. Children with speech sound disorder continue to use immature phonological simplification processes past the age when most children can produce words clearly.

Most speech sounds should be produced clearly and most words should be pronounced accurately according to age and community norms by age 7 years. The most frequently misarticulated sounds also tend to be learned later, leading them to be called the "late eight" (*l, r, s, z, th, ch, dzh,* and *zh*). Misarticulation of any of these sounds by itself could be considered within normal limits up to age 8 years. When multiple sounds are involved, it may be appropriate to target some of those sounds as part of a plan to improve intelligibility prior to the age at which almost all children can produce them accurately. Lisping (i.e., misarticulating sibilants) is particularly common and may involve frontal or lateral patterns of airstream direction. It may be associated with an abnormal tongue-thrust swallowing pattern.

Most children with speech sound disorder respond well to treatment, and speech difficulties improve over time, and thus the disorder may not be lifelong. However, when a language disorder is also present, the speech disorder has a poorer prognosis and may be associated with specific learning disorders.

# Differential Diagnosis

**Normal variations in speech.**  Regional, social, or cultural/ethnic variations of speech should be considered before making the diagnosis.

**Hearing or other sensory impairment.**  Hearing impairment or deafness may result in abnormalities of speech. Deficits of speech sound production may be associated with a hearing impairment, other sensory deficit, or a speech-motor deficit. When speech deficits are in excess of those usually associated with these problems, a diagnosis of speech sound disorder may be made.

**Structural deficits.**   Speech impairment may be due to structural deficits (e.g., cleft palate).

**Dysarthria.**   Speech impairment may be attributable to a motor disorder, such as cerebral palsy. Neurological signs, as well as distinctive features of voice, differentiate dysarthria from speech sound disorder, although in young children (under 3 years) differentiation may be difficult, particularly when there is no or minimal general body motor involvement (as in, e.g., Worster-Drought syndrome).

**Selective mutism.**   Limited use of speech may be a sign of selective mutism, an anxiety disorder that is characterized by a lack of speech in one or more contexts or settings. Selective mutism may develop in children with a speech disorder because of embarassment about their impairments, but many children with selective mutism exhibit normal speech in "safe" settings, such as at home or with close friends.

# Childhood-Onset Fluency Disorder (Stuttering)

Diagnostic Criteria                                              **315.35** (F80.81)

A. Disturbances in the normal fluency and time patterning of speech that are inappropriate for the individual's age and language skills, persist over time, and are characterized by frequent and marked occurrences of one (or more) of the following:
   1. Sound and syllable repetitions.
   2. Sound prolongations of consonants as well as vowels.
   3. Broken words (e.g., pauses within a word).
   4. Audible or silent blocking (filled or unfilled pauses in speech).
   5. Circumlocutions (word substitutions to avoid problematic words).
   6. Words produced with an excess of physical tension.
   7. Monosyllabic whole-word repetitions (e.g., "I-I-I-I see him").
B. The disturbance causes anxiety about speaking or limitations in effective communication, social participation, or academic or occupational performance, individually or in any combination.
C. The onset of symptoms is in the early developmental period. (**Note:** Later-onset cases are diagnosed as 307.0 [F98.5] adult-onset fluency disorder.)
D. The disturbance is not attributable to a speech-motor or sensory deficit, dysfluency associated with neurological insult (e.g., stroke, tumor, trauma), or another medical condition and is not better explained by another mental disorder.

## Diagnostic Features

The essential feature of childhood-onset fluency disorder (stuttering) is a disturbance in the normal fluency and time patterning of speech that is inappropriate for the individual's age. This disturbance is characterized by frequent repetitions or prolongations of sounds or syllables and by other types of speech dysfluencies, including broken words (e.g., pauses within a word), audible or silent blocking (i.e., filled or unfilled pauses in speech), circumlocutions (i.e., word substitutions to avoid problematic words), words produced with an excess of physical tension, and monosyllabic whole-word repetitions (e.g., "I-I-I-I see him"). The disturbance in fluency interferes with academic or occupational achievement or with social communication. The extent of the disturbance varies from situation to situation and often is more severe when there is special pressure to communicate (e.g., giving a report at school, interviewing for a job). Dysfluency is often absent during oral reading, singing, or talking to inanimate objects or to pets.

## Associated Features Supporting Diagnosis

Fearful anticipation of the problem may develop. The speaker may attempt to avoid dysfluencies by linguistic mechanisms (e.g., altering the rate of speech, avoiding certain words or sounds) or by avoiding certain speech situations, such as telephoning or public speaking. In addition to being features of the condition, stress and anxiety have been shown to exacerbate dysfluency.

Childhood-onset fluency disorder may also be accompanied by motor movements (e.g., eye blinks, tics, tremors of the lips or face, jerking of the head, breathing movements, fist clenching). Children with fluency disorder show a range of language abilities, and the relationship between fluency disorder and language abilities is unclear.

## Development and Course

Childhood-onset fluency disorder, or developmental stuttering, occurs by age 6 for 80%–90% of affected individuals, with age at onset ranging from 2 to 7 years. The onset can be insidious or more sudden. Typically, dysfluencies start gradually, with repetition of initial consonants, first words of a phrase, or long words. The child may not be aware of dysfluencies. As the disorder progresses, the dysfluencies become more frequent and interfering, occurring on the most meaningful words or phrases in the utterance. As the child becomes aware of the speech difficulty, he or she may develop mechanisms for avoiding the dysfluencies and emotional responses, including avoidance of public speaking and use of short and simple utterances. Longitudinal research shows that 65%–85% of children recover from the dysfluency, with severity of fluency disorder at age 8 years predicting recovery or persistence into adolescence and beyond.

## Risk and Prognostic Factors

**Genetic and physiological.**   The risk of stuttering among first-degree biological relatives of individuals with childhood-onset fluency disorder is more than three times the risk in the general population.

## Functional Consequences of Childhood-Onset Fluency Disorder (Stuttering)

In addition to being features of the condition, stress and anxiety can exacerbate dysfluency. Impairment of social functioning may result from this anxiety.

## Differential Diagnosis

**Sensory deficits.**   Dysfluencies of speech may be associated with a hearing impairment or other sensory deficit or a speech-motor deficit. When the speech dysfluencies are in excess of those usually associated with these problems, a diagnosis of childhood-onset fluency disorder may be made.

**Normal speech dysfluencies.**   The disorder must be distinguished from normal dysfluencies that occur frequently in young children, which include whole-word or phrase repetitions (e.g., "I want, I want ice cream"), incomplete phrases, interjections, unfilled pauses, and parenthetical remarks. If these difficulties increase in frequency or complexity as the child grows older, a diagnosis of childhood-onset fluency disorder is appropriate.

**Medication side effects.**   Stuttering may occur as a side effect of medication and may be detected by a temporal relationship with exposure to the medication.

**Adult-onset dysfluencies.**   If onset of dysfluencies is during or after adolescence, it is an "adult-onset dysfluency" rather than a neurodevelopmental disorder. Adult-onset dysfluencies are associated with specific neurological insults and a variety of medical conditions and mental disorders and may be specified with them, but they are not a DSM-5 diagnosis.

**Tourette's disorder.**   Vocal tics and repetitive vocalizations of Tourette's disorder should be distinguishable from the repetitive sounds of childhood-onset fluency disorder by their nature and timing.

# Social (Pragmatic) Communication Disorder

| Diagnostic Criteria | 315.39 (F80.89) |
|---|---|

A. Persistent difficulties in the social use of verbal and nonverbal communication as manifested by all of the following:

1. Deficits in using communication for social purposes, such as greeting and sharing information, in a manner that is appropriate for the social context.
2. Impairment of the ability to change communication to match context or the needs of the listener, such as speaking differently in a classroom than on a playground, talking differently to a child than to an adult, and avoiding use of overly formal language.
3. Difficulties following rules for conversation and storytelling, such as taking turns in conversation, rephrasing when misunderstood, and knowing how to use verbal and nonverbal signals to regulate interaction.
4. Difficulties understanding what is not explicitly stated (e.g., making inferences) and nonliteral or ambiguous meanings of language (e.g., idioms, humor, metaphors, multiple meanings that depend on the context for interpretation).

B. The deficits result in functional limitations in effective communication, social participation, social relationships, academic achievement, or occupational performance, individually or in combination.

C. The onset of the symptoms is in the early developmental period (but deficits may not become fully manifest until social communication demands exceed limited capacities).

D. The symptoms are not attributable to another medical or neurological condition or to low abilities in the domains of word structure and grammar, and are not better explained by autism spectrum disorder, intellectual disability (intellectual developmental disorder), global developmental delay, or another mental disorder.

## Diagnostic Features

Social (pragmatic) communication disorder is characterized by a primary difficulty with pragmatics, or the social use of language and communication, as manifested by deficits in understanding and following social rules of verbal and nonverbal communication in naturalistic contexts, changing language according to the needs of the listener or situation, and following rules for conversations and storytelling. The deficits in social communication result in functional limitations in effective communication, social participation, development of social relationships, academic achievement, or occupational performance. The deficits are not better explained by low abilities in the domains of structural language or cognitive ability.

## Associated Features Supporting Diagnosis

The most common associated feature of social (pragmatic) communication disorder is language impairment, which is characterized by a history of delay in reaching language milestones, and historical, if not current, structural language problems (see "Language Disorder" earlier in this chapter). Individuals with social communication deficits may avoid social interactions. Attention-deficit/hyperactivity disorder (ADHD), behavioral problems, and specific learning disorders are also more common among affected individuals.

## Development and Course

Because social (pragmatic) communication depends on adequate developmental progress in speech and language, diagnosis of social (pragmatic) communication disorder is rare among children younger than 4 years. By age 4 or 5 years, most children should possess adequate speech and language abilities to permit identification of specific deficits in social communication. Milder forms of the disorder may not become apparent until early adolescence, when language and social interactions become more complex.

The outcome of social (pragmatic) communication disorder is variable, with some children improving substantially over time and others continuing to have difficulties persisting into adulthood. Even among those who have significant improvements, the early deficits in pragmatics may cause lasting impairments in social relationships and behavior and also in acquisition of other related skills, such as written expression.

## Risk and Prognostic Factors

**Genetic and physiological.**   A family history of autism spectrum disorder, communication disorders, or specific learning disorder appears to increase the risk for social (pragmatic) communication disorder.

## Differential Diagnosis

**Autism spectrum disorder.**    Autism spectrum disorder is the primary diagnostic consideration for individuals presenting with social communication deficits. The two disorders can be differentiated by the presence in autism spectrum disorder of restricted/repetitive patterns of behavior, interests, or activities and their absence in social (pragmatic) communication disorder. Individuals with autism spectrum disorder may only display the restricted/repetitive patterns of behavior, interests, and activities during the early developmental period, so a comprehensive history should be obtained. Current absence of symptoms would not preclude a diagnosis of autism spectrum disorder, if the restricted interests and repetitive behaviors were present in the past. A diagnosis of social (pragmatic) communication disorder should be considered only if the developmental history fails to reveal any evidence of restricted/repetitive patterns of behavior, interests, or activities.

**Attention-deficit/hyperactivity disorder.**    Primary deficits of ADHD may cause impairments in social communication and functional limitations of effective communication, social participation, or academic achievement.

**Social anxiety disorder (social phobia).**    The symptoms of social communication disorder overlap with those of social anxiety disorder. The differentiating feature is the timing of the onset of symptoms. In social (pragmatic) communication disorder, the individual has never had effective social communication; in social anxiety disorder, the social communication skills developed appropriately but are not utilized because of anxiety, fear, or distress about social interactions.

**Intellectual disability (intellectual developmental disorder) and global developmental delay.**    Social communication skills may be deficient among individuals with global developmental delay or intellectual disability, but a separate diagnosis is not given unless the social communication deficits are clearly in excess of the intellectual limitations.

# Unspecified Communication Disorder

## 307.9 (F80.9)

This category applies to presentations in which symptoms characteristic of communication disorder that cause clinically significant distress or impairment in social, occupational, or other important areas of functioning predominate but do not meet the full criteria for communication disorder or for any of the disorders in the neurodevelopmental disorders diagnostic class. The unspecified communication disorder category is used in situations in which the clinician chooses *not* to specify the reason that the criteria are not met for communication disorder or for a specific neurodevelopmental disorder, and includes presentations in which there is insufficient information to make a more specific diagnosis.

# Autism Spectrum Disorder

## Autism Spectrum Disorder

Diagnostic Criteria                                              **299.00 (F84.0)**

A. Persistent deficits in social communication and social interaction across multiple contexts, as manifested by the following, currently or by history (examples are illustrative, not exhaustive; see text):

1. Deficits in social-emotional reciprocity, ranging, for example, from abnormal social approach and failure of normal back-and-forth conversation; to reduced sharing of interests, emotions, or affect; to failure to initiate or respond to social interactions.
2. Deficits in nonverbal communicative behaviors used for social interaction, ranging, for example, from poorly integrated verbal and nonverbal communication; to abnormalities in eye contact and body language or deficits in understanding and use of gestures; to a total lack of facial expressions and nonverbal communication.
3. Deficits in developing, maintaining, and understanding relationships, ranging, for example, from difficulties adjusting behavior to suit various social contexts; to difficulties in sharing imaginative play or in making friends; to absence of interest in peers.

*Specify* current severity:

**Severity is based on social communication impairments and restricted, repetitive patterns of behavior** (see Table 2).

B. Restricted, repetitive patterns of behavior, interests, or activities, as manifested by at least two of the following, currently or by history (examples are illustrative, not exhaustive; see text):

1. Stereotyped or repetitive motor movements, use of objects, or speech (e.g., simple motor stereotypies, lining up toys or flipping objects, echolalia, idiosyncratic phrases).
2. Insistence on sameness, inflexible adherence to routines, or ritualized patterns of verbal or nonverbal behavior (e.g., extreme distress at small changes, difficulties with transitions, rigid thinking patterns, greeting rituals, need to take same route or eat same food every day).
3. Highly restricted, fixated interests that are abnormal in intensity or focus (e.g., strong attachment to or preoccupation with unusual objects, excessively circumscribed or perseverative interests).
4. Hyper- or hyporeactivity to sensory input or unusual interest in sensory aspects of the environment (e.g., apparent indifference to pain/temperature, adverse response to specific sounds or textures, excessive smelling or touching of objects, visual fascination with lights or movement).

*Specify* current severity:

**Severity is based on social communication impairments and restricted, repetitive patterns of behavior** (see Table 2).

C. Symptoms must be present in the early developmental period (but may not become fully manifest until social demands exceed limited capacities, or may be masked by learned strategies in later life).

D. Symptoms cause clinically significant impairment in social, occupational, or other important areas of current functioning.

E. These disturbances are not better explained by intellectual disability (intellectual developmental disorder) or global developmental delay. Intellectual disability and autism spectrum disorder frequently co-occur; to make comorbid diagnoses of autism spectrum disorder and intellectual disability, social communication should be below that expected for general developmental level.

**Note:** Individuals with a well-established DSM-IV diagnosis of autistic disorder, Asperger's disorder, or pervasive developmental disorder not otherwise specified should be given the diagnosis of autism spectrum disorder. Individuals who have marked deficits in social communication, but whose symptoms do not otherwise meet criteria for autism spectrum disorder, should be evaluated for social (pragmatic) communication disorder.

*Specify* if:

**With or without accompanying intellectual impairment**

**With or without accompanying language impairment**

**Associated with a known medical or genetic condition or environmental factor** (**Coding note:** Use additional code to identify the associated medical or genetic condition.)

**Associated with another neurodevelopmental, mental, or behavioral disorder** (**Coding note:** Use additional code[s] to identify the associated neurodevelopmental, mental, or behavioral disorder[s].)

**With catatonia** (refer to the criteria for catatonia associated with another mental disorder, [DSM-5] pp. 119–120, for definition) (**Coding note:** Use additional code 293.89 [F06.1] catatonia associated with autism spectrum disorder to indicate the presence of the comorbid catatonia.)

# Recording Procedures

For autism spectrum disorder that is associated with a known medical or genetic condition or environmental factor, or with another neurodevelopmental, mental, or behavioral disorder, record autism spectrum disorder associated with (name of condition, disorder, or factor) (e.g., autism spectrum disorder associated with Rett syndrome). Severity should be recorded as level of support needed for each of the two psychopathological domains in Table 2 (e.g., "requiring very substantial support for deficits in social communication and requiring substantial support for restricted, repetitive behaviors"). Specification of "with accompanying intellectual impairment" or "without accompanying intellectual impairment" should be recorded next. Language impairment specification should be recorded thereafter. If there is accompanying language impairment, the current level of verbal functioning should be recorded (e.g., "with accompanying language impairment—no intelligible speech" or "with accompanying language impairment—phrase speech"). If catatonia is present, record separately "catatonia associated with autism spectrum disorder."

**TABLE 2  Severity levels for autism spectrum disorder**

| Severity level | Social communication | Restricted, repetitive behaviors |
|---|---|---|
| Level 3 "Requiring very substantial support" | Severe deficits in verbal and nonverbal social communication skills cause severe impairments in functioning, very limited initiation of social interactions, and minimal response to social overtures from others. For example, a person with few words of intelligible speech who rarely initiates interaction and, when he or she does, makes unusual approaches to meet needs only and responds to only very direct social approaches. | Inflexibility of behavior, extreme difficulty coping with change, or other restricted/repetitive behaviors markedly interfere with functioning in all spheres. Great distress/difficulty changing focus or action. |
| Level 2 "Requiring substantial support" | Marked deficits in verbal and nonverbal social communication skills; social impairments apparent even with supports in place; limited initiation of social interactions; and reduced or abnormal responses to social overtures from others. For example, a person who speaks simple sentences, whose interaction is limited to narrow special interests, and who has markedly odd nonverbal communication. | Inflexibility of behavior, difficulty coping with change, or other restricted/repetitive behaviors appear frequently enough to be obvious to the casual observer and interfere with functioning in a variety of contexts. Distress and/or difficulty changing focus or action. |
| Level 1 "Requiring support" | Without supports in place, deficits in social communication cause noticeable impairments. Difficulty initiating social interactions, and clear examples of atypical or unsuccessful responses to social overtures of others. May appear to have decreased interest in social interactions. For example, a person who is able to speak in full sentences and engages in communication but whose to-and-fro conversation with others fails, and whose attempts to make friends are odd and typically unsuccessful. | Inflexibility of behavior causes significant interference with functioning in one or more contexts. Difficulty switching between activities. Problems of organization and planning hamper independence. |

## Specifiers

The severity specifiers (see Table 2) may be used to describe succinctly the current symptomatology (which might fall below level 1), with the recognition that severity may vary by context and fluctuate over time. Severity of social communication difficulties and restricted, repetitive behaviors should be separately rated. The descriptive severity categories should not be used to determine eligibility for and provision of services; these can only be developed at an individual level and through discussion of personal priorities and targets.

Regarding the specifier "with or without accompanying intellectual impairment," understanding the (often uneven) intellectual profile of a child or adult with autism spectrum disorder is necessary for interpreting diagnostic features. Separate estimates of verbal and nonverbal skill are necessary (e.g., using untimed nonverbal tests to assess potential strengths in individuals with limited language).

To use the specifier "with or without accompanying language impairment," the current level of verbal functioning should be assessed and described. Examples of the specific descriptions for "with accompanying language impairment" might include no intelligible speech (nonverbal), single words only, or phrase speech. Language level in individuals "without accompanying language impairment" might be further described by speaks in full sentences or has fluent speech. Since receptive language may lag behind expressive language development in autism spectrum disorder, receptive and expressive language skills should be considered separately.

The specifier "associated with a known medical or genetic condition or environmental factor" should be used when the individual has a known genetic disorder (e.g., Rett syndrome, fragile X syndrome, Down syndrome), a medical disorder (e.g. epilepsy), or a history of environmental exposure (e.g., valproate, fetal alcohol syndrome, very low birth weight).

Additional neurodevelopmental, mental or behavioral conditions should also be noted (e.g., attention-deficit/hyperactivity disorder; developmental coordination disorder; disruptive behavior, impulse-control, or conduct disorders; anxiety, depressive, or bipolar disorders; tics or Tourette's disorder; self-injury; feeding, elimination, or sleep disorders).

## Diagnostic Features

The essential features of autism spectrum disorder are persistent impairment in reciprocal social communication and social interaction (Criterion A), and restricted, repetitive patterns of behavior, interests, or activities (Criterion B). These symptoms are present from early childhood and limit or impair everyday functioning (Criteria C and D). The stage at which functional impairment becomes obvious will vary according to characteristics of the individual and his or her environment. Core diagnostic features are evident in the developmental period, but intervention, compensation, and current supports may mask difficulties in at least some contexts. Manifestations of the disorder also vary greatly depending on the severity of the autistic condition, developmental level, and chronological age; hence, the term *spectrum*. Autism spectrum disorder encompasses disorders previously referred to as early infantile autism, childhood autism, Kanner's autism, high-functioning autism, atypical autism, pervasive developmental disorder not otherwise specified, childhood disintegrative disorder, and Asperger's disorder.

The impairments in communication and social interaction specified in Criterion A are pervasive and sustained. Diagnoses are most valid and reliable when based on multiple sources of information, including clinician's observations, caregiver history, and, when possible, self-report. Verbal and nonverbal deficits in social communication have varying manifestations, depending on the individual's age, intellectual level, and language ability, as well as other factors such as treatment history and current support. Many individuals have language deficits, ranging from complete lack of speech through language delays, poor comprehension of speech, echoed speech, or stilted and overly literal language. Even when formal language skills (e.g., vocabulary, grammar) are intact, the use of language for reciprocal social communication is impaired in autism spectrum disorder.

Deficits in social-emotional reciprocity (i.e., the ability to engage with others and share thoughts and feelings) are clearly evident in young children with the disorder, who may show little or no initiation of social interaction and no sharing of emotions, along with reduced or absent imitation of others' behavior. What language exists is often one-sided, lacking in social reciprocity, and used to request or label rather than to comment, share feelings, or converse. In adults without intellectual disabilities or language delays, deficits in social-emotional reciprocity may be most apparent in difficulties processing and responding to complex social cues (e.g., when and how to join a conversation, what not to say). Adults who have developed compensation strategies for some social challenges still struggle in novel or unsupported situations and suffer from the effort and anxiety of consciously calculating what is socially intuitive for most individuals.

Deficits in nonverbal communicative behaviors used for social interaction are manifested by absent, reduced, or atypical use of eye contact (relative to cultural norms), gestures, facial expressions, body orientation, or speech intonation. An early feature of autism spectrum disorder is impaired joint attention as manifested by a lack of pointing, showing, or bringing objects to share interest with others, or failure to follow someone's pointing or eye gaze. Individuals may learn a few functional gestures, but their repertoire is smaller than that of others, and they often fail to use expressive gestures spontaneously in communication. Among adults with fluent language, the difficulty in coordinating nonverbal communication with speech may give the impression of odd, wooden, or exaggerated "body language" during interactions. Impairment may be relatively subtle within individual modes (e.g., someone may have relatively good eye contact when speaking) but noticeable in poor integration of eye contact, gesture, body posture, prosody, and facial expression for social communication.

Deficits in developing, maintaining, and understanding relationships should be judged against norms for age, gender, and culture. There may be absent, reduced, or atypical social interest, manifested by rejection of others, passivity, or inappropriate approaches that seem aggressive or disruptive. These difficulties are particularly evident in young children, in whom there is often a lack of shared social play and imagination (e.g., age-appropriate flexible pretend play) and, later, insistence on playing by very fixed rules. Older individuals may struggle to understand what behavior is considered appropriate in one situation but not another (e.g., casual behavior during a job interview), or the different ways that language may be used to communicate (e.g., irony, white lies). There may be an apparent preference for solitary activities or for interacting with much younger or older people. Frequently, there is a desire to establish friendships without a complete or realistic idea of what friendship entails (e.g., one-sided friendships or friendships based solely on shared special interests). Relationships with siblings, co-workers, and caregivers are also important to consider (in terms of reciprocity).

Autism spectrum disorder is also defined by restricted, repetitive patterns of behavior, interests, or activities (as specified in Criterion B), which show a range of manifestations according to age and ability, intervention, and current supports. Stereotyped or repetitive behaviors include simple motor stereotypies (e.g., hand flapping, finger flicking), repetitive use of objects (e.g., spinning coins, lining up toys), and repetitive speech (e.g., echolalia, the delayed or immediate parroting of heard words; use of "you" when referring to self; stereotyped use of words, phrases, or prosodic patterns). Excessive adherence to routines and restricted patterns of behavior may be manifest in resistance to change (e.g., distress at apparently small changes, such as in packaging of a favorite food; insistence on adherence to rules; rigidity of thinking) or ritualized patterns of verbal or nonverbal behavior (e.g., repetitive questioning, pacing a perimeter). Highly restricted, fixated interests in autism spectrum disorder tend to be abnormal in intensity or focus (e.g., a toddler strongly attached to a pan; a child preoccupied with vacuum cleaners; an adult spending hours writing out timetables). Some fascinations and routines may relate to apparent hyper- or hyporeactivity to sensory input, manifested through extreme responses to specific sounds or textures, excessive smelling or touching of objects, fascination with lights or spinning objects, and sometimes apparent indifference to pain, heat, or cold. Extreme reaction to or rituals involving taste, smell, texture, or appearance of food or excessive food restrictions are common and may be a presenting feature of autism spectrum disorder.

Many adults with autism spectrum disorder without intellectual or language disabilities learn to suppress repetitive behavior in public. Special interests may be a source of pleasure and motivation and provide avenues for education and employment later in life. Diagnostic criteria may be met when restricted, repetitive patterns of behavior, interests, or activities were clearly present during childhood or at some time in the past, even if symptoms are no longer present.

Criterion D requires that the features must cause clinically significant impairment in social, occupational, or other important areas of current functioning. Criterion E specifies that the social communication deficits, although sometimes accompanied by intellectual disability (intellectual developmental disorder), are not in line with the individual's developmental level; impairments exceed difficulties expected on the basis of developmental level.

Standardized behavioral diagnostic instruments with good psychometric properties, including caregiver interviews, questionnaires and clinician observation measures, are available and can improve reliability of diagnosis over time and across clinicians.

## Associated Features Supporting Diagnosis

Many individuals with autism spectrum disorder also have intellectual impairment and/or language impairment (e.g., slow to talk, language comprehension behind production). Even those with average or high intelligence have an uneven profile of abilities. The gap between intellectual and adaptive functional skills is often large. Motor deficits are often present, including odd gait, clumsiness, and other abnormal motor signs (e.g., walking on tiptoes). Self-injury (e.g., head banging, biting the wrist) may occur, and disruptive/challenging behaviors are more common in children and adolescents with autism spectrum disorder than other disorders, including intellectual disability. Adolescents and adults with autism spectrum disorder are prone to anxiety and depression. Some individuals develop catatonic-like motor behavior (slowing and "freezing" mid-action), but these are typically not of the magnitude of a catatonic episode. However, it is possible for individuals with autism spectrum disorder to experience a marked deterioration in motor symptoms and display a full catatonic episode with symptoms such as mutism, posturing, grimacing and waxy flexibility. The risk period for comorbid catatonia appears to be greatest in the adolescent years.

## Prevalence

In recent years, reported frequencies for autism spectrum disorder across U.S. and non-U.S. countries have approached 1% of the population, with similar estimates in child and adult samples. It remains unclear whether higher rates reflect an expansion of the diagnostic criteria of DSM-IV to include subthreshold cases, increased awareness, differences in study methodology, or a true increase in the frequency of autism spectrum disorder.

## Development and Course

The age and pattern of onset also should be noted for autism spectrum disorder. Symptoms are typically recognized during the second year of life (12–24 months of age) but may be seen earlier than 12 months if developmental delays are severe, or noted later than 24 months if symptoms are more subtle. The pattern of onset description might include information about early developmental delays or any losses of social or language skills. In cases where skills have been lost, parents or caregivers may give a history of a gradual or relatively rapid deterioration in social behaviors or language skills. Typically, this would occur between 12 and 24 months of age and is distinguished from the rare instances of developmental regression occurring after at least 2 years of normal development (previously described as childhood disintegrative disorder).

The behavioral features of autism spectrum disorder first become evident in early childhood, with some cases presenting a lack of interest in social interaction in the first year of life. Some children with autism spectrum disorder experience developmental plateaus or regression, with a gradual or relatively rapid deterioration in social behaviors or use of language, often during the first 2 years of life. Such losses are rare in other disorders and may be a useful "red flag" for autism spectrum disorder. Much more unusual and warranting more extensive medical investigation are losses of skills beyond social communication (e.g., loss of self-care, toileting, motor skills) or those occurring after the second birthday (see also Rett syndrome in the section "Differential Diagnosis" for this disorder).

First symptoms of autism spectrum disorder frequently involve delayed language development, often accompanied by lack of social interest or unusual social interactions (e.g., pulling individuals by the hand without any attempt to look at them), odd play patterns (e.g., carrying toys around but never playing with them), and unusual communication patterns (e.g., knowing the alphabet but not responding to own name). Deafness may be suspected but is typically ruled out. During the second year, odd and repetitive behaviors and the absence of typical play become more apparent. Since many typically developing young children have strong preferences and enjoy repetition (e.g., eating the same foods, watching the same video multiple times), distinguishing restricted and repetitive behaviors that are diagnostic of autism spectrum disorder can be difficult in preschoolers. The clinical distinction is based on the type, frequency, and intensity of the behavior (e.g., a child who daily lines up objects for hours and is very distressed if any item is moved).

Autism spectrum disorder is not a degenerative disorder, and it is typical for learning and compensation to continue throughout life. Symptoms are often most marked in early childhood and early school years, with developmental gains typical in later childhood in at least some areas (e.g., increased interest in social interaction). A small proportion of individuals deteriorate behaviorally during adolescence, whereas most others improve. Only a minority of individuals with autism spectrum disorder live and work independently in adulthood; those who do tend to have superior language and intellectual abilities and are able to find a niche that matches their special interests and skills. In general, individuals with lower levels of impairment may be better able to function independently. However, even these individuals may remain socially naive and vulnerable, have difficulties organizing practical demands without aid, and are prone to anxiety and depression. Many adults report using compensation strategies and coping mechanisms to mask their difficulties in public but suffer from the stress and effort of maintaining a socially acceptable facade. Scarcely anything is known about old age in autism spectrum disorder.

Some individuals come for first diagnosis in adulthood, perhaps prompted by the diagnosis of autism in a child in the family or a breakdown of relations at work or home. Obtaining detailed developmental history in such cases may be difficult, and it is important to consider self-reported difficulties. Where clinical observation suggests criteria are currently met, autism spectrum disorder may be diagnosed, provided there is no evidence of good social and communication skills in childhood. For example, the report (by parents or another relative) that the individual had ordinary and sustained reciprocal friendships and good nonverbal communication skills throughout childhood would rule out a diagnosis of autism spectrum disorder; however, the absence of developmental information in itself should not do so.

Manifestations of the social and communication impairments and restricted/repetitive behaviors that define autism spectrum disorder are clear in the developmental period. In later life, intervention or compensation, as well as current supports, may mask these difficulties in at least some contexts. However, symptoms remain sufficient to cause current impairment in social, occupational, or other important areas of functioning.

# Risk and Prognostic Factors

The best established prognostic factors for individual outcome within autism spectrum disorder are presence or absence of associated intellectual disability and language impairment (e.g., functional language by age 5 years is a good prognostic sign) and additional mental health problems. Epilepsy, as a comorbid diagnosis, is associated with greater intellectual disability and lower verbal ability.

**Environmental.**  A variety of nonspecific risk factors, such as advanced parental age, low birth weight, or fetal exposure to valproate, may contribute to risk of autism spectrum disorder.

**Genetic and physiological.**  Heritability estimates for autism spectrum disorder have ranged from 37% to higher than 90%, based on twin concordance rates. Currently, as many as 15% of cases of autism spectrum disorder appear to be associated with a known genetic mutation, with different de novo copy number variants or de novo mutations in specific genes associated with the disorder in different families. However, even when an autism spectrum disorder is associated with a known genetic mutation, it does not appear to be fully penetrant. Risk for the remainder of cases appears to be polygenic, with perhaps hundreds of genetic loci making relatively small contributions.

# Culture-Related Diagnostic Issues

Cultural differences will exist in norms for social interaction, nonverbal communication, and relationships, but individuals with autism spectrum disorder are markedly impaired against the norms for their cultural context. Cultural and socioeconomic factors may affect age at recognition or diagnosis; for example, in the United States, late or underdiagnosis of autism spectrum disorder among African American children may occur.

# Gender-Related Diagnostic Issues

Autism spectrum disorder is diagnosed four times more often in males than in females. In clinic samples, females tend to be more likely to show accompanying intellectual disability, suggesting that girls without accompanying intellectual impairments or language delays may go unrecognized, perhaps because of subtler manifestation of social and communication difficulties.

# Functional Consequences of Autism Spectrum Disorder

In young children with autism spectrum disorder, lack of social and communication abilities may hamper learning, especially learning through social interaction or in settings with peers. In the home, insistence on routines and aversion to change, as well as sensory sensitivities, may interfere with eating and sleeping and make routine care (e.g., haircuts, dental work) extremely difficult. Adaptive skills are typically below measured IQ. Extreme difficulties in planning, organization, and coping with change negatively impact academic achievement, even for students with above-average intelligence. During adulthood, these individuals may have difficulties establishing independence because of continued rigidity and difficulty with novelty.

Many individuals with autism spectrum disorder, even without intellectual disability, have poor adult psychosocial functioning as indexed by measures such as independent living and gainful employment. Functional consequences in old age are unknown, but social isolation and communication problems (e.g., reduced help-seeking) are likely to have consequences for health in older adulthood.

## Differential Diagnosis

**Rett syndrome.**   Disruption of social interaction may be observed during the regressive phase of Rett syndrome (typically between 1–4 years of age); thus, a substantial proportion of affected young girls may have a presentation that meets diagnostic criteria for autism spectrum disorder. However, after this period, most individuals with Rett syndrome improve their social communication skills, and autistic features are no longer a major area of concern. Consequently, autism spectrum disorder should be considered only when all diagnostic criteria are met.

**Selective mutism.**   In selective mutism, early development is not typically disturbed. The affected child usually exhibits appropriate communication skills in certain contexts and settings. Even in settings where the child is mute, social reciprocity is not impaired, nor are restricted or repetitive patterns of behavior present.

**Language disorders and social (pragmatic) communication disorder.**   In some forms of language disorder, there may be problems of communication and some secondary social difficulties. However, specific language disorder is not usually associated with abnormal nonverbal communication, nor with the presence of restricted, repetitive patterns of behavior, interests, or activities.

When an individual shows impairment in social communication and social interactions but does not show restricted and repetitive behavior or interests, criteria for social (pragmatic) communication disorder, instead of autism spectrum disorder, may be met. The diagnosis of autism spectrum disorder supersedes that of social (pragmatic) communication disorder whenever the criteria for autism spectrum disorder are met, and care should be taken to inquire carefully regarding past or current restricted/repetitive behavior.

**Intellectual disability (intellectual developmental disorder) without autism spectrum disorder.**   Intellectual disability without autism spectrum disorder may be difficult to differentiate from autism spectrum disorder in very young children. Individuals with intellectual disability who have not developed language or symbolic skills also present a challenge for differential diagnosis, since repetitive behavior often occurs in such individuals as well. A diagnosis of autism spectrum disorder in an individual with intellectual disability is appropriate when social communication and interaction are significantly impaired relative to the developmental level of the individual's nonverbal skills (e.g., fine motor skills, nonverbal problem solving). In contrast, intellectual disability is the appropriate diagnosis when there is no apparent discrepancy between the level of social-communicative skills and other intellectual skills.

**Stereotypic movement disorder.**   Motor stereotypies are among the diagnostic characteristics of autism spectrum disorder, so an additional diagnosis of stereotypic movement disorder is not given when such repetitive behaviors are better explained by the presence of autism spectrum disorder. However, when stereotypies cause self-injury and become a focus of treatment, both diagnoses may be appropriate.

**Attention-deficit/hyperactivity disorder.**   Abnormalities of attention (overly focused or easily distracted) are common in individuals with autism spectrum disorder, as is hyperactivity. A diagnosis of attention-deficit/hyperactivity disorder (ADHD) should be considered when attentional difficulties or hyperactivity exceeds that typically seen in individuals of comparable mental age.

**Schizophrenia.**   Schizophrenia with childhood onset usually develops after a period of normal, or near normal, development. A prodromal state has been described in which social impairment and atypical interests and beliefs occur, which could be confused with the social deficits seen in autism spectrum disorder. Hallucinations and delusions, which are defining features of schizophrenia, are not features of autism spectrum disorder. However, clinicians must take into account the potential for individuals with autism spectrum disorder to be concrete in their interpretation of questions regarding the key features of schizophrenia (e.g., "Do you hear voices when no one is there?" "Yes [on the radio]").

## Comorbidity

Autism spectrum disorder is frequently associated with intellectual impairment and structural language disorder (i.e., an inability to comprehend and construct sentences with proper grammar), which should be noted under the relevant specifiers when applicable. Many individuals with autism spectrum disorder have psychiatric symptoms that do not form part of the diagnostic criteria for the disorder (about 70% of individuals with autism spectrum disorder may have one comorbid mental disorder, and 40% may have two or more comorbid mental disorders). When criteria for both ADHD and autism spectrum disorder are met, both diagnoses should be given. This same principle applies to concurrent diagnoses of autism spectrum disorder and developmental coordination disorder, anxiety disorders, depressive disorders, and other comorbid diagnoses. Among individuals who are nonverbal or have language deficits, observable signs such as changes in sleep or eating and increases in challenging behavior should trigger an evaluation for anxiety or depression. Specific learning difficulties (literacy and numeracy) are common, as is developmental coordination disorder. Medical conditions commonly associated with autism spectrum disorder should be noted under the "associated with a known medical or genetic condition or environmental factor" specifier. Such medical conditions include epilepsy, sleep problems, and constipation. Avoidant/restrictive food intake disorder is a fairly frequent presenting feature of autism spectrum disorder, and extreme and narrow food preferences may persist.

# Attention-Deficit/Hyperactivity Disorder

## Attention-Deficit/Hyperactivity Disorder

### Diagnostic Criteria

A. A persistent pattern of inattention and/or hyperactivity-impulsivity that interferes with functioning or development, as characterized by (1) and/or (2):

1. **Inattention:** Six (or more) of the following symptoms have persisted for at least 6 months to a degree that is inconsistent with developmental level and that negatively impacts directly on social and academic/occupational activities:

   **Note:** The symptoms are not solely a manifestation of oppositional behavior, defiance, hostility, or failure to understand tasks or instructions. For older adolescents and adults (age 17 and older), at least five symptoms are required.

   a. Often fails to give close attention to details or makes careless mistakes in schoolwork, at work, or during other activities (e.g., overlooks or misses details, work is inaccurate).

   b. Often has difficulty sustaining attention in tasks or play activities (e.g., has difficulty remaining focused during lectures, conversations, or lengthy reading).

   c. Often does not seem to listen when spoken to directly (e.g., mind seems elsewhere, even in the absence of any obvious distraction).

   d. Often does not follow through on instructions and fails to finish schoolwork, chores, or duties in the workplace (e.g., starts tasks but quickly loses focus and is easily sidetracked).

   e. Often has difficulty organizing tasks and activities (e.g., difficulty managing sequential tasks; difficulty keeping materials and belongings in order; messy, disorganized work; has poor time management; fails to meet deadlines).

   f. Often avoids, dislikes, or is reluctant to engage in tasks that require sustained mental effort (e.g., schoolwork or homework; for older adolescents and adults, preparing reports, completing forms, reviewing lengthy papers).

   g. Often loses things necessary for tasks or activities (e.g., school materials, pencils, books, tools, wallets, keys, paperwork, eyeglasses, mobile telephones).

   h. Is often easily distracted by extraneous stimuli (for older adolescents and adults, may include unrelated thoughts).

   i. Is often forgetful in daily activities (e.g., doing chores, running errands; for older adolescents and adults, returning calls, paying bills, keeping appointments).

2. **Hyperactivity and impulsivity:** Six (or more) of the following symptoms have persisted for at least 6 months to a degree that is inconsistent with developmental level and that negatively impacts directly on social and academic/occupational activities:

   **Note:** The symptoms are not solely a manifestation of oppositional behavior, defiance, hostility, or a failure to understand tasks or instructions. For older adolescents and adults (age 17 and older), at least five symptoms are required.

    a. Often fidgets with or taps hands or feet or squirms in seat.

    b. Often leaves seat in situations when remaining seated is expected (e.g., leaves his or her place in the classroom, in the office or other workplace, or in other situations that require remaining in place).

    c. Often runs about or climbs in situations where it is inappropriate. (**Note:** In adolescents or adults, may be limited to feeling restless.)

    d. Often unable to play or engage in leisure activities quietly.

    e. Is often "on the go," acting as if "driven by a motor" (e.g., is unable to be or uncomfortable being still for extended time, as in restaurants, meetings; may be experienced by others as being restless or difficult to keep up with).

    f. Often talks excessively.

    g. Often blurts out an answer before a question has been completed (e.g., completes people's sentences; cannot wait for turn in conversation).

    h. Often has difficulty waiting his or her turn (e.g., while waiting in line).

    i. Often interrupts or intrudes on others (e.g., butts into conversations, games, or activities; may start using other people's things without asking or receiving permission; for adolescents and adults, may intrude into or take over what others are doing).

B. Several inattentive or hyperactive-impulsive symptoms were present prior to age 12 years.

C. Several inattentive or hyperactive-impulsive symptoms are present in two or more settings (e.g., at home, school, or work; with friends or relatives; in other activities).

D. There is clear evidence that the symptoms interfere with, or reduce the quality of, social, academic, or occupational functioning.

E. The symptoms do not occur exclusively during the course of schizophrenia or another psychotic disorder and are not better explained by another mental disorder (e.g., mood disorder, anxiety disorder, dissociative disorder, personality disorder, substance intoxication or withdrawal).

*Specify* whether:

    **314.01 (F90.2) Combined presentation:** If both Criterion A1 (inattention) and Criterion A2 (hyperactivity-impulsivity) are met for the past 6 months.

    **314.00 (F90.0) Predominantly inattentive presentation:** If Criterion A1 (inattention) is met but Criterion A2 (hyperactivity-impulsivity) is not met for the past 6 months.

    **314.01 (F90.1) Predominantly hyperactive/impulsive presentation:** If Criterion A2 (hyperactivity-impulsivity) is met and Criterion A1 (inattention) is not met for the past 6 months.

*Specify* if:

    **In partial remission:** When full criteria were previously met, fewer than the full criteria have been met for the past 6 months, and the symptoms still result in impairment in social, academic, or occupational functioning.

*Specify* current severity:

    **Mild:** Few, if any, symptoms in excess of those required to make the diagnosis are present, and symptoms result in no more than minor impairments in social or occupational functioning.

    **Moderate:** Symptoms or functional impairment between "mild" and "severe" are present.

**Severe:** Many symptoms in excess of those required to make the diagnosis, or several symptoms that are particularly severe, are present, or the symptoms result in marked impairment in social or occupational functioning.

## Diagnostic Features

The essential feature of attention-deficit/hyperactivity disorder (ADHD) is a persistent pattern of inattention and/or hyperactivity-impulsivity that interferes with functioning or development. *Inattention* manifests behaviorally in ADHD as wandering off task, lacking persistence, having difficulty sustaining focus, and being disorganized and is not due to defiance or lack of comprehension. *Hyperactivity* refers to excessive motor activity (such as a child running about) when it is not appropriate, or excessive fidgeting, tapping, or talkativeness. In adults, hyperactivity may manifest as extreme restlessness or wearing others out with their activity. *Impulsivity* refers to hasty actions that occur in the moment without forethought and that have high potential for harm to the individual (e.g., darting into the street without looking). Impulsivity may reflect a desire for immediate rewards or an inability to delay gratification. Impulsive behaviors may manifest as social intrusiveness (e.g., interrupting others excessively) and/or as making important decisions without consideration of long-term consequences (e.g., taking a job without adequate information).

ADHD begins in childhood. The requirement that several symptoms be present before age 12 years conveys the importance of a substantial clinical presentation during childhood. At the same time, an earlier age at onset is not specified because of difficulties in establishing precise childhood onset retrospectively. Adult recall of childhood symptoms tends to be unreliable, and it is beneficial to obtain ancillary information.

Manifestations of the disorder must be present in more than one setting (e.g., home and school, work). Confirmation of substantial symptoms across settings typically cannot be done accurately without consulting informants who have seen the individual in those settings. Typically, symptoms vary depending on context within a given setting. Signs of the disorder may be minimal or absent when the individual is receiving frequent rewards for appropriate behavior, is under close supervision, is in a novel setting, is engaged in especially interesting activities, has consistent external stimulation (e.g., via electronic screens), or is interacting in one-on-one situations (e.g., the clinician's office).

## Associated Features Supporting Diagnosis

Mild delays in language, motor, or social development are not specific to ADHD but often co-occur. Associated features may include low frustration tolerance, irritability, or mood lability. Even in the absence of a specific learning disorder, academic or work performance is often impaired. Inattentive behavior is associated with various underlying cognitive processes, and individuals with ADHD may exhibit cognitive problems on tests of attention, executive function, or memory, although these tests are not sufficiently sensitive or specific to serve as diagnostic indices. By early adulthood, ADHD is associated with an increased risk of suicide attempt, primarily when comorbid with mood, conduct, or substance use disorders.

No biological marker is diagnostic for ADHD. As a group, compared with peers, children with ADHD display increased slow wave electroencephalograms, reduced total brain volume on magnetic resonance imaging, and possibly a delay in posterior to anterior cortical maturation, but these findings are not diagnostic. In the uncommon cases where there is a known genetic cause (e.g., fragile X syndrome, 22q11 deletion syndrome), the ADHD presentation should still be diagnosed.

## Prevalence

Population surveys suggest that ADHD occurs in most cultures in about 5% of children and about 2.5% of adults.

## Development and Course

Many parents first observe excessive motor activity when the child is a toddler, but symptoms are difficult to distinguish from highly variable normative behaviors before age 4 years. ADHD is most often identified during elementary school years, and inattention becomes more prominent and impairing. The disorder is relatively stable through early adolescence, but some individuals have a worsened course with development of antisocial behaviors. In most individuals with ADHD, symptoms of motoric hyperactivity become less obvious in adolescence and adulthood, but difficulties with restlessness, inattention, poor planning, and impulsivity persist. A substantial proportion of children with ADHD remain relatively impaired into adulthood.

In preschool, the main manifestation is hyperactivity. Inattention becomes more prominent during elementary school. During adolescence, signs of hyperactivity (e.g., running and climbing) are less common and may be confined to fidgetiness or an inner feeling of jitteriness, restlessness, or impatience. In adulthood, along with inattention and restlessness, impulsivity may remain problematic even when hyperactivity has diminished.

## Risk and Prognostic Factors

**Temperamental.** ADHD is associated with reduced behavioral inhibition, effortful control, or constraint; negative emotionality; and/or elevated novelty seeking. These traits may predispose some children to ADHD but are not specific to the disorder.

**Environmental.** Very low birth weight (less than 1,500 grams) conveys a two- to three-fold risk for ADHD, but most children with low birth weight do not develop ADHD. Although ADHD is correlated with smoking during pregnancy, some of this association reflects common genetic risk. A minority of cases may be related to reactions to aspects of diet. There may be a history of child abuse, neglect, multiple foster placements, neurotoxin exposure (e.g., lead), infections (e.g., encephalitis), or alcohol exposure in utero. Exposure to environmental toxicants has been correlated with subsequent ADHD, but it is not known whether these associations are causal.

**Genetic and physiological.** ADHD is elevated in the first-degree biological relatives of individuals with ADHD. The heritability of ADHD is substantial. While specific genes have been correlated with ADHD, they are neither necessary nor sufficient causal factors. Visual and hearing impairments, metabolic abnormalities, sleep disorders, nutritional deficiencies, and epilepsy should be considered as possible influences on ADHD symptoms.

ADHD is not associated with specific physical features, although rates of minor physical anomalies (e.g., hypertelorism, highly arched palate, low-set ears) may be relatively elevated. Subtle motor delays and other neurological soft signs may occur. (Note that marked co-occurring clumsiness and motor delays should be coded separately [e.g., developmental coordination disorder].)

**Course modifiers.**   Family interaction patterns in early childhood are unlikely to cause ADHD but may influence its course or contribute to secondary development of conduct problems.

## Culture-Related Diagnostic Issues

Differences in ADHD prevalence rates across regions appear attributable mainly to different diagnostic and methodological practices. However, there also may be cultural variation in attitudes toward or interpretations of children's behaviors. Clinical identification rates in the United States for African American and Latino populations tend to be lower than for Caucasian populations. Informant symptom ratings may be influenced by cultural group of the child and the informant, suggesting that culturally appropriate practices are relevant in assessing ADHD.

## Gender-Related Diagnostic Issues

ADHD is more frequent in males than in females in the general population, with a ratio of approximately 2:1 in children and 1.6:1 in adults. Females are more likely than males to present primarily with inattentive features.

## Functional Consequences of Attention-Deficit/Hyperactivity Disorder

ADHD is associated with reduced school performance and academic attainment, social rejection, and, in adults, poorer occupational performance, attainment, attendance, and higher probability of unemployment as well as elevated interpersonal conflict. Children with ADHD are significantly more likely than their peers without ADHD to develop conduct disorder in adolescence and antisocial personality disorder in adulthood, consequently increasing the likelihood for substance use disorders and incarceration. The risk of subsequent substance use disorders is elevated, especially when conduct disorder or antisocial personality disorder develops. Individuals with ADHD are more likely than peers to be injured. Traffic accidents and violations are more frequent in drivers with ADHD. There may be an elevated likelihood of obesity among individuals with ADHD.

Inadequate or variable self-application to tasks that require sustained effort is often interpreted by others as laziness, irresponsibility, or failure to cooperate. Family relationships may be characterized by discord and negative interactions. Peer relationships are often disrupted by peer rejection, neglect, or teasing of the individual with ADHD. On average, individuals with ADHD obtain less schooling, have poorer vocational achievement, and have reduced intellectual scores than their peers, although there is great variability. In its severe form, the disorder is markedly impairing, affecting social, familial, and scholastic/occupational adjustment.

Academic deficits, school-related problems, and peer neglect tend to be most associated with elevated symptoms of inattention, whereas peer rejection and, to a lesser extent, accidental injury are most salient with marked symptoms of hyperactivity or impulsivity.

## Differential Diagnosis

**Oppositional defiant disorder.**   Individuals with oppositional defiant disorder may resist work or school tasks that require self-application because they resist conforming to others' demands. Their behavior is characterized by negativity, hostility, and defiance. These symptoms must be differentiated from aversion to school or mentally demanding tasks due to difficulty in sustaining mental effort, forgetting instructions, and impulsivity in individuals with ADHD. Complicating the differential diagnosis is the fact that some individuals with ADHD may develop secondary oppositional attitudes toward such tasks and devalue their importance.

**Intermittent explosive disorder.**   ADHD and intermittent explosive disorder share high levels of impulsive behavior. However, individuals with intermittent explosive disorder show serious aggression toward others, which is not characteristic of ADHD, and they do not experience problems with sustaining attention as seen in ADHD. In addition, intermittent explosive disorder is rare in childhood. Intermittent explosive disorder may be diagnosed in the presence of ADHD.

**Other neurodevelopmental disorders.**   The increased motoric activity that may occur in ADHD must be distinguished from the repetitive motor behavior that characterizes stereotypic movement disorder and some cases of autism spectrum disorder. In stereotypic movement disorder, the motoric behavior is generally fixed and repetitive (e.g., body rocking, self-biting), whereas the fidgetiness and restlessness in ADHD are typically generalized and not characterized by repetitive stereotypic movements. In Tourette's disorder, frequent multiple tics can be mistaken for the generalized fidgetiness of ADHD. Prolonged observation may be needed to differentiate fidgetiness from bouts of multiple tics.

**Specific learning disorder.**   Children with specific learning disorder may appear inattentive because of frustration, lack of interest, or limited ability. However, inattention in individuals with a specific learning disorder who do not have ADHD is not impairing outside of academic work.

**Intellectual disability (intellectual developmental disorder).**   Symptoms of ADHD are common among children placed in academic settings that are inappropriate to their intellectual ability. In such cases, the symptoms are not evident during nonacademic tasks. A diagnosis of ADHD in intellectual disability requires that inattention or hyperactivity be excessive for mental age.

**Autism spectrum disorder.**   Individuals with ADHD and those with autism spectrum disorder exhibit inattention, social dysfunction, and difficult-to-manage behavior. The social dysfunction and peer rejection seen in individuals with ADHD must be distinguished from the social disengagement, isolation, and indifference to facial and tonal communication cues seen in individuals with autism spectrum disorder. Children with autism spectrum disorder may display tantrums because of an inability to tolerate a change from their expected course of events. In contrast, children with ADHD may misbehave or have a tantrum during a major transition because of impulsivity or poor self-control.

**Reactive attachment disorder.**   Children with reactive attachment disorder may show social disinhibition, but not the full ADHD symptom cluster, and display other features such as a lack of enduring relationships that are not characteristic of ADHD.

**Anxiety disorders.**   ADHD shares symptoms of inattention with anxiety disorders. Individuals with ADHD are inattentive because of their attraction to external stimuli, new activities, or preoccupation with enjoyable activities. This is distinguished from the inattention due to worry and rumination seen in anxiety disorders. Restlessness might be seen in anxiety disorders. However, in ADHD, the symptom is not associated with worry and rumination.

**Depressive disorders.**   Individuals with depressive disorders may present with inability to concentrate. However, poor concentration in mood disorders becomes prominent only during a depressive episode.

**Bipolar disorder.**   Individuals with bipolar disorder may have increased activity, poor concentration, and increased impulsivity, but these features are episodic, occurring several days at a time. In bipolar disorder, increased impulsivity or inattention is accompanied by elevated mood, grandiosity, and other specific bipolar features. Children with ADHD may show significant changes in mood within the same day; such lability is distinct from a manic episode, which must last 4 or more days to be a clinical indicator of bipolar disorder, even in children. Bipolar disorder is rare in preadolescents, even when severe irritability and anger are prominent, whereas ADHD is common among children and adolescents who display excessive anger and irritability.

**Disruptive mood dysregulation disorder.**   Disruptive mood dysregulation disorder is characterized by pervasive irritability, and intolerance of frustration, but impulsiveness and disorganized attention are not essential features. However, most children and adolescents with the disorder have symptoms that also meet criteria for ADHD, which is diagnosed separately.

**Substance use disorders.**   Differentiating ADHD from substance use disorders may be problematic if the first presentation of ADHD symptoms follows the onset of abuse or frequent use. Clear evidence of ADHD before substance misuse from informants or previous records may be essential for differential diagnosis.

**Personality disorders.**   In adolescents and adults, it may be difficult to distinguish ADHD from borderline, narcissistic, and other personality disorders. All these disorders tend to share the features of disorganization, social intrusiveness, emotional dysregulation, and cognitive dysregulation. However, ADHD is not characterized by fear of abandonment, self-injury, extreme ambivalence, or other features of personality disorder. It may take extended clinical observation, informant interview, or detailed history to distinguish impulsive, socially intrusive, or inappropriate behavior from narcissistic, aggressive, or domineering behavior to make this differential diagnosis.

**Psychotic disorders.**   ADHD is not diagnosed if the symptoms of inattention and hyperactivity occur exclusively during the course of a psychotic disorder.

**Medication-induced symptoms of ADHD.**   Symptoms of inattention, hyperactivity, or impulsivity attributable to the use of medication (e.g., bronchodilators, isoniazid, neuroleptics [resulting in akathisia], thyroid replacement medication) are diagnosed as other specified or unspecified other (or unknown) substance–related disorders.

**Neurocognitive disorders.**   Early major neurocognitive disorder (dementia) and/or mild neurocognitive disorder are not known to be associated with ADHD but may present with similar clinical features. These conditions are distinguished from ADHD by their late onset.

## Comorbidity

In clinical settings, comorbid disorders are frequent in individuals whose symptoms meet criteria for ADHD. In the general population, oppositional defiant disorder co-occurs with ADHD in approximately half of children with the combined presentation and about a quarter with the predominantly inattentive presentation. Conduct disorder co-occurs in about a quarter of children or adolescents with the combined presentation, depending on age and setting. Most children and adolescents with disruptive mood dysregulation disorder have symptoms that also meet criteria for ADHD; a lesser percentage of children with ADHD have symptoms that meet criteria for disruptive mood dysregulation disorder. Specific learning disorder commonly co-occurs with ADHD. Anxiety disorders and major depressive disorder occur in a minority of individuals with ADHD but more often than in the general population. Intermittent explosive disorder occurs in a minority of adults with ADHD, but at rates above population levels. Although substance use disorders are relatively more frequent among adults with ADHD in the general population, the disorders are present in only a minority of adults with ADHD. In adults, antisocial and other personality disorders may co-occur with ADHD. Other disorders that may co-occur with ADHD include obsessive-compulsive disorder, tic disorders, and autism spectrum disorder.

# Other Specified Attention-Deficit/ Hyperactivity Disorder

### 314.01 (F90.8)

This category applies to presentations in which symptoms characteristic of attention-deficit/hyperactivity disorder that cause clinically significant distress or impairment in social, occupational or other important areas of functioning predominate but do not meet the full criteria for attention-deficit/hyperactivity disorder or any of the disorders in the neurodevelopmental disorders diagnostic class. The other specified attention-deficit/hyperactivity disorder category is used in situations in which the clinician chooses to communicate the specific reason that the presentation does not meet the criteria for attention-deficit/hyperactivity disorder or any specific neurodevelopmental disorder. This is done by recording "other specified attention-deficit/hyperactivity disorder" followed by the specific reason (e.g., "with insufficient inattention symptoms").

# Unspecified Attention-Deficit/Hyperactivity Disorder

## 314.01 (F90.9)

This category applies to presentations in which symptoms characteristic of attention-deficit/hyperactivity disorder that cause clinically significant distress or impairment in social, occupational, or other important areas of functioning predominate but do not meet the full criteria for attention-deficit/hyperactivity disorder or any of the disorders in the neurodevelopmental disorders diagnostic class. The unspecified attention-deficit/hyperactivity disorder category is used in situations in which the clinician chooses *not* to specify the reason that the criteria are not met for attention-deficit/hyperactivity disorder or for a specific neurodevelopmental disorder, and includes presentations in which there is insufficient information to make a more specific diagnosis.

# Specific Learning Disorder

## Specific Learning Disorder

### Diagnostic Criteria

A. Difficulties learning and using academic skills, as indicated by the presence of at least one of the following symptoms that have persisted for at least 6 months, despite the provision of interventions that target those difficulties:

1. Inaccurate or slow and effortful word reading (e.g., reads single words aloud incorrectly or slowly and hesitantly, frequently guesses words, has difficulty sounding out words).
2. Difficulty understanding the meaning of what is read (e.g., may read text accurately but not understand the sequence, relationships, inferences, or deeper meanings of what is read).
3. Difficulties with spelling (e.g., may add, omit, or substitute vowels or consonants).
4. Difficulties with written expression (e.g., makes multiple grammatical or punctuation errors within sentences; employs poor paragraph organization; written expression of ideas lacks clarity).
5. Difficulties mastering number sense, number facts, or calculation (e.g., has poor understanding of numbers, their magnitude, and relationships; counts on fingers

to add single-digit numbers instead of recalling the math fact as peers do; gets lost in the midst of arithmetic computation and may switch procedures).

   6. Difficulties with mathematical reasoning (e.g., has severe difficulty applying mathematical concepts, facts, or procedures to solve quantitative problems).

B. The affected academic skills are substantially and quantifiably below those expected for the individual's chronological age, and cause significant interference with academic or occupational performance, or with activities of daily living, as confirmed by individually administered standardized achievement measures and comprehensive clinical assessment. For individuals age 17 years and older, a documented history of impairing learning difficulties may be substituted for the standardized assessment.

C. The learning difficulties begin during school-age years but may not become fully manifest until the demands for those affected academic skills exceed the individual's limited capacities (e.g., as in timed tests, reading or writing lengthy complex reports for a tight deadline, excessively heavy academic loads).

D. The learning difficulties are not better accounted for by intellectual disabilities, uncorrected visual or auditory acuity, other mental or neurological disorders, psychosocial adversity, lack of proficiency in the language of academic instruction, or inadequate educational instruction.

**Note:** The four diagnostic criteria are to be met based on a clinical synthesis of the individual's history (developmental, medical, family, educational), school reports, and psychoeducational assessment.

**Coding note:** Specify all academic domains and subskills that are impaired. When more than one domain is impaired, each one should be coded individually according to the following specifiers.

*Specify* if:

### 315.00 (F81.0) With impairment in reading:

Word reading accuracy
Reading rate or fluency
Reading comprehension

**Note:** *Dyslexia* is an alternative term used to refer to a pattern of learning difficulties characterized by problems with accurate or fluent word recognition, poor decoding, and poor spelling abilities. If dyslexia is used to specify this particular pattern of difficulties, it is important also to specify any additional difficulties that are present, such as difficulties with reading comprehension or math reasoning.

### 315.2 (F81.81) With impairment in written expression:

Spelling accuracy
Grammar and punctuation accuracy
Clarity or organization of written expression

### 315.1 (F81.2) With impairment in mathematics:

Number sense
Memorization of arithmetic facts
Accurate or fluent calculation
Accurate math reasoning

**Note:** *Dyscalculia* is an alternative term used to refer to a pattern of difficulties characterized by problems processing numerical information, learning arithmetic facts, and performing accurate or fluent calculations. If dyscalculia is used to specify this particular pattern of mathematic difficulties, it is important also to specify any additional difficulties that are present, such as difficulties with math reasoning or word reasoning accuracy.

*Specify* current severity:

**Mild:** Some difficulties learning skills in one or two academic domains, but of mild enough severity that the individual may be able to compensate or function well when provided with appropriate accommodations or support services, especially during the school years.

**Moderate:** Marked difficulties learning skills in one or more academic domains, so that the individual is unlikely to become proficient without some intervals of intensive and specialized teaching during the school years. Some accommodations or supportive services at least part of the day at school, in the workplace, or at home may be needed to complete activities accurately and efficiently.

**Severe:** Severe difficulties learning skills, affecting several academic domains, so that the individual is unlikely to learn those skills without ongoing intensive individualized and specialized teaching for most of the school years. Even with an array of appropriate accommodations or services at home, at school, or in the workplace, the individual may not be able to complete all activities efficiently.

## Recording Procedures

Each impaired academic domain and subskill of specific learning disorder should be recorded. Because of ICD coding requirements, impairments in reading, impairments in written expression, and impairments in mathematics, with their corresponding impairments in subskills, must be coded separately. For example, impairments in reading and mathematics and impairments in the subskills of reading rate or fluency, reading comprehension, accurate or fluent calculation, and accurate math reasoning would be coded and recorded as 315.00 (F81.0) specific learning disorder with impairment in reading, with impairment in reading rate or fluency and impairment in reading comprehension; 315.1 (F81.2) specific learning disorder with impairment in mathematics, with impairment in accurate or fluent calculation and impairment in accurate math reasoning.

## Diagnostic Features

Specific learning disorder is a neurodevelopmental disorder with a biological origin that is the basis for abnormalities at a cognitive level that are associated with the behavioral signs of the disorder. The biological origin includes an interaction of genetic, epigenetic, and environmental factors, which affect the brain's ability to perceive or process verbal or nonverbal information efficiently and accurately.

One essential feature of specific learning disorder is persistent difficulties learning keystone academic skills (Criterion A), with onset during the years of formal schooling (i.e., the developmental period). Key academic skills include reading of single words accurately and fluently, reading comprehension, written expression and spelling, arithmetic calculation, and mathematical reasoning (solving mathematical problems). In contrast to talking or walking, which are acquired developmental milestones that emerge with brain maturation, academic skills (e.g., reading, spelling, writing, mathematics) have to be taught and learned explicitly. Specific learning disorder disrupts the normal pattern of learning academic skills; it is not simply a consequence of lack of opportunity of learning or inadequate instruction. Difficulties mastering these key academic skills may also impede learning in other academic subjects (e.g., history, science, social studies), but those problems are attributable to difficulties learning the underlying academic skills. Difficulties learning to map letters with the sounds of one's language—to read printed words (often called *dyslexia*)—is one of the most common manifestations of specific learning disorder. The learning difficulties manifest as a range of observable, descriptive behaviors or symptoms (as listed in Criteria A1–A6). These clinical symptoms may be observed, probed by means of the clinical interview, or ascertained from school reports, rating scales, or descriptions in previous educational or psychological assessments. The learning difficulties are persistent, not transitory. In children and adolescents, *persistence* is defined as restricted progress in learning (i.e., no evidence that the individual is catching up with classmates) for at least 6 months despite the provision of extra help at home or school. For example, difficulties learning to read single words that do not fully or rapidly remit with the provision of instruction in phonological skills or word identification strategies may indicate a specific learning disorder. Evidence of persistent learning difficulties may be derived from cumulative school reports, portfolios of the child's evaluated work, curriculum-based measures, or clinical interview. In adults, persistent difficulty refers to ongoing difficulties in literacy or numeracy skills that manifest during childhood or adolescence, as indicated by cumulative evidence from school reports, evaluated portfolios of work, or previous assessments.

A second key feature is that the individual's performance of the affected academic skills is well below average for age (Criterion B). One robust clinical indicator of difficulties learning academic skills is low academic achievement for age or average achievement that is sustainable only by extraordinarily high levels of effort or support. In children, the low academic skills cause significant interference in school performance (as indicated by school reports and teacher's grades or ratings). Another clinical indicator, particularly in adults, is avoidance of activities that require the academic skills. Also in adulthood, low academic skills interfere with occupational performance or everyday activities requiring those skills (as indicated by self-report or report by others). However, this criterion also requires psychometric evidence from an individually administered, psychometrically sound and culturally appropriate test of academic achievement that is norm-referenced or criterion-referenced. Academic skills are distributed along a continuum, so there is no natural cutpoint that can be used to differentiate individuals with and without specific learning disorder. Thus, any threshold used to specify what constitutes significantly low academic achievement (e.g., academic skills well below age expectation) is to a large extent arbitrary. Low achievement scores on one or more standardized tests or subtests within an academic domain (i.e., at least 1.5 standard deviations [SD] below the population mean for age, which translates to a standard score of 78 or less, which is below the 7th percentile) are needed for the greatest diagnostic certainty. However, precise scores will vary according to the particular standardized tests that are used. On the basis of clinical judgment, a more lenient threshold may be used (e.g., 1.0–2.5 SD below the population mean for age), when learning difficulties are supported by converging evidence from clinical assessment, academic history, school reports, or test scores. Moreover, since standardized tests are not available in all languages, the diagnosis may then be based in part on clinical judgment of scores on available test measures.

A third core feature is that the learning difficulties are readily apparent in the early school years in most individuals (Criterion C). However, in others, the learning difficulties may not manifest fully until later school years, by which time learning demands have increased and exceed the individual's limited capacities.

Another key diagnostic feature is that the learning difficulties are considered "specific," for four reasons. First, they are not attributable to intellectual disabilities (intellectual disability [intellectual developmental disorder]); global developmental delay; hearing or vision disorders, or neurological or motor disorders) (Criterion D). Specific learning disorder affects learning in individuals who otherwise demonstrate normal levels of intellectual functioning (generally estimated by an IQ score of greater than about 70 [±5 points allowing for measurement error]). The phrase "unexpected academic underachievement" is often cited as the defining characteristic of specific learning disorder in that the specific learning disabilities are not part of a more general learning difficulty as manifested in intellectual disability or global developmental delay. Specific learning disorder may also occur in individuals identified as intellectually "gifted." These individuals may be able to sustain apparently adequate academic functioning by using compensatory strategies, extraordinarily high effort, or support, until the learning demands or assessment procedures (e.g., timed tests) pose barriers to their demonstrating their learning or accomplishing required tasks. Second, the learning difficulty cannot be attributed to more general external factors, such as economic or environmental disadvantage, chronic absenteeism, or lack of education as typically provided in the individual's community context. Third, the learning difficulty cannot be attributed to a neurological (e.g., pediatric stroke) or motor disorders or to vision or hearing disorders, which are often associated with problems learning academic skills but are distinguishable by presence of neurological signs. Finally, the learning difficulty may be restricted to one academic skill or domain (e.g., reading single words, retrieving or calculating number facts).

Comprehensive assessment is required. Specific learning disorder can only be diagnosed after formal education starts but can be diagnosed at any point afterward in children, adolescents, or adults, providing there is evidence of onset during the years of formal schooling (i.e., the developmental period). No single data source is sufficient for a diagnosis of specific learning disorder. Rather, specific learning disorder is a clinical diagnosis based on a synthesis of the individual's medical, developmental, educational, and family history; the history of the learning difficulty, including its previous and current manifestation; the impact of the difficulty on academic, occupational, or social functioning; previous or current school reports; portfolios of work requiring academic skills; curriculum-based assessments; and previous or current scores from individual standardized tests of academic achievement. If an intellectual, sensory, neurological, or motor disorder is suspected, then the clinical assessment for specific learning disorder should also include methods appropriate for these disorders.

Thus, comprehensive assessment will involve professionals with expertise in specific learning disorder and psychological/cognitive assessment. Since specific learning disorder typically persists into adulthood, reassessment is rarely necessary, unless indicated by marked changes in the learning difficulties (amelioration or worsening) or requested for specific purposes.

## Associated Features Supporting Diagnosis

Specific learning disorder is frequently but not invariably preceded, in preschool years, by delays in attention, language, or motor skills that may persist and co-occur with specific learning disorder. An uneven profile of abilities is common, such as above-average abilities in drawing, design, and other visuospatial abilities, but slow, effortful, and inaccurate reading and poor reading comprehension and written expression. Individuals with specific learning disorder typically (but not invariably) exhibit poor performance on psychological tests of cognitive processing. However, it remains unclear whether these cognitive abnormalities are the cause, correlate, or consequence of the learning difficulties. Also, although cognitive deficits associated with difficulties learning to read words are well documented, those associated with other manifestations of specific learning disorder (e.g., reading comprehension, arithmetic computation, written expression) are underspecified or unknown. Moreover, individuals with similar behavioral symptoms or test scores are found to have a variety of cognitive deficits, and many of these processing deficits are also found in other neurodevelopmental disorders (e.g., attention-deficit/hyperactivity disorder [ADHD], autistic spectrum disorder, communication disorders, developmental coordination disorder). Thus, assessment of cognitive processing deficits is not required for diagnostic assessment. Specific learning disorder is associated with increased risk for suicidal ideation and suicide attempts in children, adolescents, and adults.

There are no known biological markers of specific learning disorder. As a group, individuals with the disorder show circumscribed alterations in cognitive processing and brain structure and function. Genetic differences are also evident at the group level. But cognitive testing, neuroimaging, or genetic testing are not useful for diagnosis at this time.

## Prevalence

The prevalence of specific learning disorder across the academic domains of reading, writing, and mathematics is 5%–15% among school-age children across different languages and cultures. Prevalence in adults is unknown but appears to be approximately 4%.

## Development and Course

Onset, recognition, and diagnosis of specific learning disorder usually occurs during the elementary school years when children are required to learn to read, spell, write, and learn mathematics. However, precursors such as language delays or deficits, difficulties in rhyming or counting, or difficulties with fine motor skills required for writing commonly occur in early childhood before the start of formal schooling. Manifestations may be behavioral (e.g., a reluctance to engage in learning; oppositional behavior). Specific learning disorder is lifelong, but the course and clinical expression are variable, in part depending on the interactions among the task demands of the environment, the range and severity of the individual's learning difficulties, the individual's learning abilities, comorbidity, and the available support systems and intervention. Nonetheless, problems with reading fluency and comprehension, spelling, written expression, and numeracy skills in everyday life typically persist into adulthood.

Changes in manifestation of symptoms occur with age, so that an individual may have a persistent or shifting array of learning difficulties across the lifespan.

Examples of symptoms that may be observed among preschool-age children include a lack of interest in playing games with language sounds (e.g., repetition, rhyming), and they may have trouble learning nursery rhymes. Preschool children with specific learning disorder may frequently use baby talk, mispronounce words, and have trouble remembering names of letters, numbers, or days of the week. They may fail to recognize letters in their own names and have trouble learning to count. Kindergarten-age children with specific learning disorder may be unable to recognize and write letters, may be unable to write their own names, or may use invented spelling. They may have trouble breaking down spoken words into syllables (e.g., "cowboy" into "cow" and "boy") and trouble recognizing words that rhyme (e.g., cat, bat, hat). Kindergarten-age children also may have trouble connecting letters with their sounds (e.g., letter b makes the sound /b/) and may be unable to recognize phonemes (e.g., do not know which in a set of words [e.g., dog, man, car] starts with the same sound as "cat").

Specific learning disorder in elementary school–age children typically manifests as marked difficulty learning letter-sound correspondence (particularly in English-speaking children), fluent word decoding, spelling, or math facts; reading aloud is slow, inaccurate, and effortful, and some children struggle to understand the magnitude that a spoken or written number represents. Children in primary grades (grades 1–3) may continue to have problems recognizing and manipulating phonemes, be unable to read common one-syllable words (such as mat or top), and be unable recognize common irregularly spelled words (e.g., said, two). They may commit reading errors that indicate problems in connecting sounds and letters (e.g., "big" for "got") and have difficulty sequencing numbers and letters. Children in grades 1-3 also may have difficulty remembering number facts or arithmetic procedures for adding, subtracting, and so forth, and may complain that reading or arithmetic is hard and avoid doing it. Children with specific learning disorder in the middle grades (grades 4–6) may mispronounce or skip parts of long, multisyllable words (e.g., say "conible" for "convertible," "aminal" for "animal") and confuse words that sound alike (e.g., "tornado" for "volcano"). They may have trouble remembering dates, names, and telephone numbers and may have trouble completing homework or tests on time. Children in the middle grades also may have poor comprehension with or without slow, effortful, and inaccurate reading, and they may have trouble reading small function words (e.g., that, the, an, in). They may have very poor spelling and poor written work. They may get the first part of a word correctly, then guess wildly (e.g., read "clover" as "clock"), and may express fear of reading aloud or refuse to read aloud.

By contrast, adolescents may have mastered word decoding, but reading remains slow and effortful, and they are likely to show marked problems in reading comprehension and written expression (including poor spelling) and poor mastery of math facts or mathematical problem solving. During adolescence and into adulthood, individuals with specific learning disorder may continue to make numerous spelling mistakes and read single words and connected text slowly and with much effort, with trouble pronouncing multisyllable words. They may frequently need to reread material to understand or get the main point and have trouble making inferences from written text. Adolescents and adults may avoid activities that demand reading or arithmetic (reading for pleasure, reading instructions). Adults with specific learning disorder have ongoing spelling problems, slow and effortful reading, or problems making important inferences from numerical information in work-related written documents. They may avoid both leisure and work-related activities that demand reading or writing or use alternative approaches to access print (e.g., text-to-speech/ speech-to-text software, audiobooks, audiovisual media).

An alternative clinical expression is that of circumscribed learning difficulties that persist across the lifespan, such as an inability to master the basic sense of number (e.g., to know which of a pair of numbers or dots represents the larger magnitude), or lack of proficiency in word identification or spelling. Avoidance of or reluctance to engage in activities requiring academic skills is common in children, adolescents, and adults. Episodes of severe anxiety or anxiety disorders, including somatic complaints or panic attacks, are common across the lifespan and accompany both the circumscribed and the broader expression of learning difficulties.

## Risk and Prognostic Factors

**Environmental.**    Prematurity or very low birth weight increases the risk for specific learning disorder, as does prenatal exposure to nicotine.

**Genetic and physiological.**    Specific learning disorder appears to aggregate in families, particularly when affecting reading, mathematics, and spelling. The relative risk of specific learning disorder in reading or mathematics is substantially higher (e.g., 4– 8 times and 5–10 times higher, respectively) in first-degree relatives of individuals with these learning difficulties compared with those without them. Family history of reading difficulties (dyslexia) and parental literacy skills predict literacy problems or specific learning disorder in offspring, indicating the combined role of genetic and environmental factors.

There is high heritability for both reading ability and reading disability in alphabetic and nonalphabetic languages, including high heritability for most manifestations of learning abilities and disabilities (e.g., heritability estimate values greater than 0.6). Covariation between various manifestations of learning difficulties is high, suggesting that genes related to one presentation are highly correlated with genes related to another manifestation.

**Course modifiers.**    Marked problems with inattentive behavior in preschool years is predictive of later difficulties in reading and mathematics (but not necessarily specific learning disorder) and nonresponse to effective academic interventions. Delay or disorders in speech or language, or impaired cognitive processing (e.g., phonological awareness, working memory, rapid serial naming) in preschool years, predicts later specific learning disorder in reading and written expression. Comorbidity with ADHD is predictive of worse mental health outcome than that associated with specific learning disorder without ADHD. Systematic, intensive, individualized instruction, using evidence-based interventions, may improve or ameliorate the learning difficulties in some individuals or promote the use of compensatory strategies in others, thereby mitigating the otherwise poor outcomes.

## Culture-Related Diagnostic Issues

Specific learning disorder occurs across languages, cultures, races, and socioeconomic conditions but may vary in its manifestation according to the nature of the spoken and written symbol systems and cultural and educational practices. For example, the cognitive processing requirements of reading and of working with numbers vary greatly across orthographies. In the English language, the observable hallmark clinical symptom of difficulties learning to read is inaccurate and slow reading of single words; in other alphabetic languages that have more direct mapping between sounds and letters (e.g., Spanish, German) and in non-alphabetic languages (e.g., Chinese, Japanese), the hallmark feature is slow but accurate reading. In English-language learners, assessment should include consideration of whether the source of reading difficulties is a limited proficiency with English or a specific learning disorder. Risk factors for specific learning disorder in English-language learners include a family history of specific learning disorder or language delay in the native language, as well as learning difficulties in English and failure to catch up with peers. If there is suspicion of cultural or language differences (e.g., as in an English-language learner), the assessment needs to take into account the individual's language proficiency in his or her first or native language as well as in the second language (in this example, English). Also, assessment should consider the linguistic and cultural context in which the individual is living, as well as his or her educational and learning history in the original culture and language.

## Gender-Related Diagnostic Issues

Specific learning disorder is more common in males than in females (ratios range from about 2:1 to 3:1) and cannot be attributed to factors such as ascertainment bias, definitional or measurement variation, language, race, or socioeconomic status.

## Functional Consequences of Specific Learning Disorder

Specific learning disorder can have negative functional consequences across the lifespan, including lower academic attainment, higher rates of high school dropout, lower rates of postsecondary education, high levels of psychological distress and poorer overall mental health, higher rates of unemployment and under-employment, and lower incomes. School dropout and co-occurring depressive symptoms increase the risk for poor mental health outcomes, including suicidality, whereas high levels of social or emotional support predict better mental health outcomes.

# Differential Diagnosis

**Normal variations in academic attainment.**   Specific learning disorder is distinguished from normal variations in academic attainment due to external factors (e.g., lack of educational opportunity, consistently poor instruction, learning in a second language), because the learning difficulties persist in the presence of adequate educational opportunity and exposure to the same instruction as the peer group, and competency in the language of instruction, even when it is different from one's primary spoken language.

**Intellectual disability (intellectual developmental disorder).**   Specific learning disorder differs from general learning difficulties associated with intellectual disability, because the learning difficulties occur in the presence of normal levels of intellectual functioning (i.e., IQ score of at least 70 ± 5). If intellectual disability is present, specific learning disorder can be diagnosed only when the learning difficulties are in excess of those usually associated with the intellectual disability.

**Learning difficulties due to neurological or sensory disorders.**   Specific learning disorder is distinguished from learning difficulties due to neurological or sensory disorders (e.g., pediatric stroke, traumatic brain injury, hearing impairment, vision impairment), because in these cases there are abnormal findings on neurological examination.

**Neurocognitive disorders.**   Specific learning disorder is distinguished from learning problems associated with neurodegenerative cognitive disorders, because in specific learning disorder the clinical expression of specific learning difficulties occurs during the developmental period, and the difficulties do not manifest as a marked decline from a former state.

**Attention-deficit/hyperactivity disorder.**   Specific learning disorder is distinguished from the poor academic performance associated with ADHD, because in the latter condition the problems may not necessarily reflect specific difficulties in learning academic skills but rather may reflect difficulties in performing those skills. However, the co-occurrence of specific learning disorder and ADHD is more frequent than expected by chance. If criteria for both disorders are met, both diagnoses can be given.

**Psychotic disorders.**   Specific learning disorder is distinguished from the academic and cognitive-processing difficulties associated with schizophrenia or psychosis, because with these disorders there is a decline (often rapid) in these functional domains.

# Comorbidity

Specific learning disorder commonly co-occurs with neurodevelopmental (e.g., ADHD, communication disorders, developmental coordination disorder, autistic spectrum disorder) or other mental disorders (e.g., anxiety disorders, depressive and bipolar disorders). These comorbidities do not necessarily exclude the diagnosis specific learning disorder but may make testing and differential diagnosis more difficult, because each of the co-occurring disorders independently interferes with the execution of activities of daily living, including learning. Thus, clinical judgment is required to attribute such impairment to learning difficulties. If there is an indication that another diagnosis could account for the difficulties learning keystone academic skills described in Criterion A, specific learning disorder should not be diagnosed.

# Motor Disorders

## Developmental Coordination Disorder

Diagnostic Criteria                                                    **315.4** (F82)

A. The acquisition and execution of coordinated motor skills is substantially below that expected given the individual's chronological age and opportunity for skill learning and use. Difficulties are manifested as clumsiness (e.g., dropping or bumping into objects) as well as slowness and inaccuracy of performance of motor skills (e.g., catching an object, using scissors or cutlery, handwriting, riding a bike, or participating in sports).

B. The motor skills deficit in Criterion A significantly and persistently interferes with activities of daily living appropriate to chronological age (e.g., self-care and self-maintenance) and impacts academic/school productivity, prevocational and vocational activities, leisure, and play.

C. Onset of symptoms is in the early developmental period.

D. The motor skills deficits are not better explained by intellectual disability (intellectual developmental disorder) or visual impairment and are not attributable to a neurological condition affecting movement (e.g., cerebral palsy, muscular dystrophy, degenerative disorder).

## Diagnostic Features

The diagnosis of developmental coordination disorder is made by a clinical synthesis of the history (developmental and medical), physical examination, school or workplace report, and individual assessment using psychometrically sound and culturally appropriate standardized tests. The manifestation of impaired skills requiring motor coordination (Criterion A) varies with age. Young children may be delayed in achieving motor milestones (i.e., sitting, crawling, walking), although many achieve typical motor milestones. They also may be delayed in developing skills such as negotiating stairs, pedaling, buttoning shirts, completing puzzles, and using zippers. Even when the skill is achieved, movement execution may appear awkward, slow, or less precise than that of peers. Older children and adults may display slow speed or inaccuracy with motor aspects of activities such as assembling puzzles, building models, playing ball games (especially in teams), handwriting, typing, driving, or carrying out self-care skills.

Developmental coordination disorder is diagnosed only if the impairment in motor skills significantly interferes with the performance of, or participation in, daily activities in family, social, school, or community life (Criterion B). Examples of such activities include getting dressed, eating meals with age-appropriate utensils and without mess, engaging in physical games with others, using specific tools in class such as rulers and scissors, and participating in team exercise activities at school. Not only is ability to perform these actions impaired, but also marked slowness in execution is common. Handwriting competence is frequently affected, consequently affecting legibility and/or speed of written output and affecting academic achievement (the impact is distinguished from specific learning difficulty by the emphasis on the motoric component of written output skills). In adults, everyday skills in education and work, especially those in which speed and accuracy are required, are affected by coordination problems.

Criterion C states that the onset of symptoms of developmental coordination disorder must be in the early developmental period. However, developmental coordination disorder is typically not diagnosed before age 5 years because there is considerable variation in the age at acquisition of many motor skills or a lack of stability of measurement in early childhood (e.g., some children catch up) or because other causes of motor delay may not have fully manifested.

Criterion D specifies that the diagnosis of developmental coordination disorder is made if the coordination difficulties are not better explained by visual impairment or attributable to a neurological condition. Thus, visual function examination and neurological examination must be included in the diagnostic evaluation. If intellectual disability (intellectual developmental disorder) is present, the motor difficulties are in excess of those expected for the mental age; however, no IQ cut-off or discrepancy criterion is specified.

Developmental coordination disorder does not have discrete subtypes; however, individuals may be impaired predominantly in gross motor skills or in fine motor skills, including handwriting skills.

Other terms used to describe developmental coordination disorder include *childhood dyspraxia, specific developmental disorder of motor function,* and *clumsy child syndrome.*

## Associated Features Supporting Diagnosis

Some children with developmental coordination disorder show additional (usually suppressed) motor activity, such as choreiform movements of unsupported limbs or mirror movements. These "overflow" movements are referred to as *neurodevelopmental immaturities* or *neurological soft signs* rather than neurological abnormalities. In both current literature and clinical practice, their role in diagnosis is still unclear, requiring further evaluation.

## Prevalence

The prevalence of developmental coordination disorder in children ages 5–11 years is 5%–6% (in children age 7 years, 1.8% are diagnosed with severe developmental coordination disorder and 3% with probable developmental coordination disorder). Males are more often affected than females, with a male:female ratio between 2:1 and 7:1.

# Development and Course

The course of developmental coordination disorder is variable but stable at least to 1 year follow-up. Although there may be improvement in the longer term, problems with coordinated movements continue through adolescence in an estimated 50%–70% of children. Onset is in early childhood. Delayed motor milestones may be the first signs, or the disorder is first recognized when the child attempts tasks such as holding a knife and fork, buttoning clothes, or playing ball games. In middle childhood, there are difficulties with motor aspects of assembling puzzles, building models, playing ball, and handwriting, as well as with organizing belongings, when motor sequencing and coordination are required. In early adulthood, there is continuing difficulty in learning new tasks involving complex/automatic motor skills, including driving and using tools. Inability to take notes and handwrite quickly may affect performance in the workplace. Co-occurrence with other disorders (see the section "Comorbidity" for this disorder) has an additional impact on presentation, course, and outcome.

# Risk and Prognostic Factors

**Environmental.** Developmental coordination disorder is more common following prenatal exposure to alcohol and in preterm and low-birth-weight children.

**Genetic and physiological.** Impairments in underlying neurodevelopmental processes—particularly in visual-motor skills, both in visual-motor perception and spatial mentalizing—have been found and affect the ability to make rapid motoric adjustments as the complexity of the required movements increases. Cerebellar dysfunction has been proposed, but the neural basis of developmental coordination disorder remains unclear. Because of the co-occurrence of developmental coordination disorder with attention-deficit/hyperactivity disorder (ADHD), specific learning disabilities, and autism spectrum disorder, shared genetic effect has been proposed. However, consistent co-occurrence in twins appears only in severe cases.

**Course modifiers.** Individuals with ADHD and with developmental coordination disorder demonstrate more impairment than individuals with ADHD without developmental coordination disorder.

# Culture-Related Diagnostic Issues

Developmental coordination disorder occurs across cultures, races, and socioeconomic conditions. By definition, "activities of daily living" implies cultural differences necessitating consideration of the context in which the individual child is living as well as whether he or she has had appropriate opportunities to learn and practice such activities.

# Functional Consequences of Developmental Coordination Disorder

Developmental coordination disorder leads to impaired functional performance in activities of daily living (Criterion B), and the impairment is increased with co-occurring conditions. Consequences of developmental coordination disorder include reduced participation in team play and sports; poor self-esteem and sense of self-worth; emotional or behavior problems; impaired academic achievement; poor physical fitness; and reduced physical activity and obesity.

## Differential Diagnosis

**Motor impairments due to another medical condition.** Problems in coordination may be associated with visual function impairment and specific neurological disorders (e.g., cerebral palsy, progressive lesions of the cerebellum, neuromuscular disorders). In such cases, there are additional findings on neurological examination.

**Intellectual disability (intellectual developmental disorder).** If intellectual disability is present, motor competences may be impaired in accordance with the intellectual disability. However, if the motor difficulties are in excess of what could be accounted for by the intellectual disability, and criteria for developmental coordination disorder are met, developmental coordination disorder can be diagnosed as well.

**Attention-deficit/hyperactivity disorder.** Individuals with ADHD may fall, bump into objects, or knock things over. Careful observation across different contexts is required to ascertain if lack of motor competence is attributable to distractibility and impulsiveness rather than to developmental coordination disorder. If criteria for both ADHD and developmental coordination disorder are met, both diagnoses can be given.

**Autism spectrum disorder.** Individuals with autism spectrum disorder may be uninterested in participating in tasks requiring complex coordination skills, such as ball sports, which will affect test performance and function but not reflect core motor competence. Co-occurrence of developmental coordination disorder and autism spectrum disorder is common. If criteria for both disorders are met, both diagnoses can be given.

**Joint hypermobility syndrome.** Individuals with syndromes causing hyperextensible joints (found on physical examination; often with a complaint of pain) may present with symptoms similar to those of developmental coordination disorder.

## Comorbidity

Disorders that commonly co-occur with developmental coordination disorder include speech and language disorder; specific learning disorder (especially reading and writing); problems of inattention, including ADHD (the most frequent coexisting condition, with about 50% co-occurrence); autism spectrum disorder; disruptive and emotional behavior problems; and joint hypermobility syndrome. Different clusters of co-occurrence may be present (e.g., a cluster with severe reading disorders, fine motor problems, and handwriting problems; another cluster with impaired movement control and motor planning). Presence of other disorders does not exclude developmental coordination disorder but may make testing more difficult and may independently interfere with the execution of activities of daily living, thus requiring examiner judgment in ascribing impairment to motor skills.

# Stereotypic Movement Disorder

| Diagnostic Criteria | 307.3 (F98.4) |
|---|---|

A. Repetitive, seemingly driven, and apparently purposeless motor behavior (e.g., hand shaking or waving, body rocking, head banging, self-biting, hitting own body).

B. The repetitive motor behavior interferes with social, academic, or other activities and may result in self-injury.

C. Onset is in the early developmental period.

D. The repetitive motor behavior is not attributable to the physiological effects of a substance or neurological condition and is not better explained by another neurodevelopmental or mental disorder (e.g., trichotillomania [hair-pulling disorder], obsessive-compulsive disorder).

*Specify* if:

**With self-injurious behavior** (or behavior that would result in an injury if preventive measures were not used)

**Without self-injurious behavior**

*Specify* if:

**Associated with a known medical or genetic condition, neurodevelopmental disorder, or environmental factor** (e.g., Lesch-Nyhan syndrome, intellectual disability [intellectual developmental disorder], intrauterine alcohol exposure)

**Coding note:** Use additional code to identify the associated medical or genetic condition, or neurodevelopmental disorder.

*Specify* current severity:

**Mild:** Symptoms are easily suppressed by sensory stimulus or distraction.

**Moderate:** Symptoms require explicit protective measures and behavioral modification.

**Severe:** Continuous monitoring and protective measures are required to prevent serious injury.

## Recording Procedures

For stereotypic movement disorder that is associated with a known medical or genetic condition, neurodevelopmental disorder, or environmental factor, record stereotypic movement disorder associated with (name of condition, disorder, or factor) (e.g., stereotypic movement disorder associated with Lesch-Nyhan syndrome).

## Specifiers

The severity of non-self-injurious stereotypic movements ranges from mild presentations that are easily suppressed by a sensory stimulus or distraction to continuous movements that markedly interfere with all activities of daily living. Self-injurious behaviors range in severity along various dimensions, including the frequency, impact on adaptive functioning, and severity of bodily injury (from mild bruising or erythema from hitting hand against body, to lacerations or amputation of digits, to retinal detachment from head banging).

# Diagnostic Features

The essential feature of stereotypic movement disorder is repetitive, seemingly driven, and apparently purposeless motor behavior (Criterion A). These behaviors are often rhythmical movements of the head, hands, or body without obvious adaptive function. The movements may or may not respond to efforts to stop them. Among typically developing children, the repetitive movements may be stopped when attention is directed to them or when the child is distracted from performing them. Among children with neurodevelopmental disorders, the behaviors are typically less responsive to such efforts. In other cases, the individual demonstrates self-restraining behaviors (e.g., sitting on hands, wrapping arms in clothing, finding a protective device).

The repertoire of behaviors is variable; each individual presents with his or her own individually patterned, "signature" behavior. Examples of non-self-injurious stereotypic movements include, but are not limited to, body rocking, bilateral flapping or rotating hand movements, flicking or fluttering fingers in front of the face, arm waving or flapping, and head nodding. Stereotyped self-injurious behaviors include, but are not limited to, repetitive head banging, face slapping, eye poking, and biting of hands, lips, or other body parts. Eye poking is particularly concerning; it occurs more frequently among children with visual impairment. Multiple movements may be combined (e.g., cocking the head, rocking the torso, waving a small string repetitively in front of the face).

Stereotypic movements may occur many times during a day, lasting a few seconds to several minutes or longer. Frequency can vary from many occurrences in a single day to several weeks elapsing between episodes. The behaviors vary in context, occurring when the individual is engrossed in other activities, when excited, stressed, fatigued, or bored. Criterion A requires that the movements be "apparently" purposeless. However, some functions may be served by the movements. For example, stereotypic movements might reduce anxiety in response to external stressors.

Criterion B states that the stereotypic movements interfere with social, academic, or other activities and, in some children, may result in self-injury (or would if protective measures were not used). If self-injury is present, it should be coded using the specifier. Onset of stereotypic movements is in the early developmental period (Criterion C). Criterion D states that the repetitive, stereotyped behavior in stereotypic movement disorder is not attributable to the physiological effects of a substance or neurological condition and is not better explained by another neurodevelopmental or mental disorder. The presence of stereotypic movements may indicate an undetected neurodevelopmental problem, especially in children ages 1–3 years.

# Prevalence

Simple stereotypic movements (e.g., rocking) are common in young typically developing children. Complex stereotypic movements are much less common (occurring in approximately 3%–4%). Between 4% and 16% of individuals with intellectual disability (intellectual developmental disorder) engage in stereotypy and self-injury. The risk is greater in individuals with severe intellectual disability. Among individuals with intellectual disability living in residential facilities, 10%–15% may have stereotypic movement disorder with self-injury.

## Development and Course

Stereotypic movements typically begin within the first 3 years of life. Simple stereotypic movements are common in infancy and may be involved in acquisition of motor mastery. In children who develop complex motor stereotypies, approximately 80% exhibit symptoms before 24 months of age, 12% between 24 and 35 months, and 8% at 36 months or older. In most typically developing children, these movements resolve over time or can be suppressed. Onset of complex motor stereotypies may be in infancy or later in the developmental period. Among individuals with intellectual disability, the stereotyped, self-injurious behaviors may persist for years, even though the typography or pattern of self-injury may change.

## Risk and Prognostic Factors

**Environmental.**   Social isolation is a risk factor for self-stimulation that may progress to stereotypic movements with repetitive self-injury. Environmental stress may also trigger stereotypic behavior. Fear may alter physiological state, resulting in increased frequency of stereotypic behaviors.

**Genetic and physiological.**   Lower cognitive functioning is linked to greater risk for stereotypic behaviors and poorer response to interventions. Stereotypic movements are more frequent among individuals with moderate-to-severe/profound intellectual disability, who by virtue of a particular syndrome (e.g., Rett syndrome) or environmental factor (e.g., an environment with relatively insufficient stimulation) seem to be at higher risk for stereotypies. Repetitive self-injurious behavior may be a behavioral phenotype in neurogenetic syndromes. For example, in Lesch-Nyhan syndrome, there are both stereotypic dystonic movements and self-mutilation of fingers, lip biting, and other forms of self-injury unless the individual is restrained, and in Rett syndrome and Cornelia de Lange syndrome, self-injury may result from the hand-to-mouth stereotypies. Stereotypic behaviors may result from a painful medical condition (e.g., middle ear infection, dental problems, gastroesophageal reflux).

## Culture-Related Diagnostic Issues

Stereotypic movement disorder, with or without self-injury, occurs in all races and cultures. Cultural attitudes toward unusual behaviors may result in delayed diagnosis. Overall cultural tolerance and attitudes toward stereotypic movement vary and must be considered.

## Differential Diagnosis

**Normal development.**   Simple stereotypic movements are common in infancy and early childhood. Rocking may occur in the transition from sleep to awake, a behavior that usually resolves with age. Complex stereotypies are less common in typically developing children and can usually be suppressed by distraction or sensory stimulation. The individual's daily routine is rarely affected, and the movements generally do not cause the child distress. The diagnosis would not be appropriate in these circumstances.

**Autism spectrum disorder.** Stereotypic movements may be a presenting symptom of autism spectrum disorder and should be considered when repetitive movements and behaviors are being evaluated. Deficits of social communication and reciprocity manifesting in autism spectrum disorder are generally absent in stereotypic movement disorder, and thus social interaction, social communication, and rigid repetitive behaviors and interests are distinguishing features. When autism spectrum disorder is present, stereotypic movement disorder is diagnosed only when there is self-injury or when the stereotypic behaviors are sufficiently severe to become a focus of treatment.

**Tic disorders.** Typically, stereotypies have an earlier age at onset (before 3 years) than do tics, which have a mean age at onset of 5–7 years. They are consistent and fixed in their pattern or topography compared with tics, which are variable in their presentation. Stereotypies may involve arms, hands, or the entire body, while tics commonly involve eyes, face, head, and shoulders. Stereotypies are more fixed, rhythmic, and prolonged in duration than tics, which, generally, are brief, rapid, random, and fluctuating. Tics and stereotypic movements are both reduced by distraction.

**Obsessive-compulsive and related disorders.** Stereotypic movement disorder is distinguished from obsessive-compulsive disorder (OCD) by the absence of obsessions, as well as by the nature of the repetitive behaviors. In OCD the individual feels driven to perform repetitive behaviors in response to an obsession or according to rules that must be applied rigidly, whereas in stereotypic movement disorder the behaviors are seemingly driven but apparently purposeless. Trichotillomania (hair-pulling disorder) and excoriation (skin-picking) disorder are characterized by body-focused repetitive behaviors (i.e., hair pulling and skin picking) that may be seemingly driven but that are not apparently purposeless, and that may not be patterned or rhythmical. Furthermore, onset in trichotillomania and excoriation disorder is not typically in the early developmental period, but rather around puberty or later.

**Other neurological and medical conditions.** The diagnosis of stereotypic movements requires the exclusion of habits, mannerisms, paroxysmal dyskinesias, and benign hereditary chorea. A neurological history and examination are required to assess features suggestive of other disorders, such as myoclonus, dystonia, tics, and chorea. Involuntary movements associated with a neurological condition may be distinguished by their signs and symptoms. For example, repetitive, stereotypic movements in tardive dyskinesia can be distinguished by a history of chronic neuroleptic use and characteristic oral or facial dyskinesia or irregular trunk or limb movements. These types of movements do not result in self-injury. A diagnosis of stereotypic movement disorder is not appropriate for repetitive skin picking or scratching associated with amphetamine intoxication or abuse (e.g., patients are diagnosed with substance/medication-induced obsessive-compulsive and related disorder) and repetitive choreoathetoid movements associated with other neurological disorders.

## Comorbidity

Stereotypic movement disorder may occur as a primary diagnosis or secondary to another disorder. For example, stereotypies are a common manifestation of a variety of neurogenetic disorders, such as Lesch-Nyhan syndrome, Rett syndrome, fragile X syndrome, Cornelia de Lange syndrome, and Smith-Magenis syndrome. When stereotypic movement disorder co-occurs with another medical condition, both should be coded.

# Tic Disorders

## Diagnostic Criteria

**Note:** A tic is a sudden, rapid, recurrent, nonrhythmic motor movement or vocalization.

**Tourette's Disorder**                                                **307.23** (F95.2)

A. Both multiple motor and one or more vocal tics have been present at some time during the illness, although not necessarily concurrently.
B. The tics may wax and wane in frequency but have persisted for more than 1 year since first tic onset.
C. Onset is before age 18 years.
D. The disturbance is not attributable to the physiological effects of a substance (e.g., cocaine) or another medical condition (e.g., Huntington's disease, postviral encephalitis).

**Persistent (Chronic) Motor or Vocal Tic Disorder**      **307.22** (F95.1)

A. Single or multiple motor or vocal tics have been present during the illness, but not both motor and vocal.
B. The tics may wax and wane in frequency but have persisted for more than 1 year since first tic onset.
C. Onset is before age 18 years.
D. The disturbance is not attributable to the physiological effects of a substance (e.g., cocaine) or another medical condition (e.g., Huntington's disease, postviral encephalitis).
E. Criteria have never been met for Tourette's disorder.

*Specify* if:
    **With motor tics only**
    **With vocal tics only**

**Provisional Tic Disorder**                                          **307.21** (F95.0)

A. Single or multiple motor and/or vocal tics.
B. The tics have been present for less than 1 year since first tic onset.
C. Onset is before age 18 years.
D. The disturbance is not attributable to the physiological effects of a substance (e.g., cocaine) or another medical condition (e.g., Huntington's disease, postviral encephalitis).
E. Criteria have never been met for Tourette's disorder or persistent (chronic) motor or vocal tic disorder.

## Specifiers

The "motor tics only" or "vocal tics only" specifier is only required for persistent (chronic) motor or vocal tic disorder.

# Diagnostic Features

Tic disorders comprise four diagnostic categories: Tourette's disorder, persistent (chronic) motor or vocal tic disorder, provisional tic disorder, and the other specified and unspecified tic disorders. Diagnosis for any tic disorder is based on the presence of motor and/or vocal tics (Criterion A), duration of tic symptoms (Criterion B), age at onset (Criterion C), and absence of any known cause such as another medical condition or substance use (Criterion D). The tic disorders are hierarchical in order (i.e., Tourette's disorder, followed by persistent [chronic] motor or vocal tic disorder, followed by provisional tic disorder, followed by the other specified and unspecified tic disorders), such that once a tic disorder at one level of the hierarchy is diagnosed, a lower hierarchy diagnosis cannot be made (Criterion E).

Tics are sudden, rapid, recurrent, nonrhythmic motor movements or vocalizations. An individual may have various tic symptoms over time, but at any point in time, the tic repertoire recurs in a characteristic fashion. Although tics can include almost any muscle group or vocalization, certain tic symptoms, such as eye blinking or throat clearing, are common across patient populations. Tics are generally experienced as involuntary but can be voluntarily suppressed for varying lengths of time.

Tics can be either simple or complex. *Simple motor tics* are of short duration (i.e., milliseconds) and can include eye blinking, shoulder shrugging, and extension of the extremities. Simple vocal tics include throat clearing, sniffing, and grunting often caused by contraction of the diaphragm or muscles of the oropharynx. *Complex motor tics* are of longer duration (i.e., seconds) and often include a combination of simple tics such as simultaneous head turning and shoulder shrugging. Complex tics can appear purposeful, such as a tic-like sexual or obscene gesture (*copropraxia*) or a tic-like imitation of someone else's movements (*echopraxia*). Similarly, complex vocal tics include repeating one's own sounds or words (*palilalia*), repeating the last-heard word or phrase (*echolalia*), or uttering socially unacceptable words, including obscenities, or ethnic, racial, or religious slurs (*coprolalia*). Importantly, coprolalia is an abrupt, sharp bark or grunt utterance and lacks the prosody of similar inappropriate speech observed in human interactions.

The presence of motor and/or vocal tics varies across the four tic disorders (Criterion A). For Tourette's disorder, both motor and vocal tics must be present, whereas for persistent (chronic) motor or vocal tic disorder, only motor or only vocal tics are present. For provisional tic disorder, motor and/or vocal tics may be present. For other specified or unspecified tic disorders, the movement disorder symptoms are best characterized as tics but are atypical in presentation or age at onset, or have a known etiology.

The 1-year minimum duration criterion (Criterion B) assures that individuals diagnosed with either Tourette's disorder or persistent (chronic) motor or vocal tic disorder have had persistent symptoms. Tics wax and wane in severity, and some individuals may have tic-free periods of weeks to months; however, an individual who has had tic symptoms of greater than 1 year's duration since first tic onset would be considered to have persistent symptoms regardless of duration of tic-free periods. For an individual with motor and/or vocal tics of less than 1 year since first tic onset, a provisional tic disorder diagnosis can be considered. There is no duration specification for other specified and unspecified tic disorders. The onset of tics must occur prior to age 18 years (Criterion C). Tic disorders typically begin in the prepubertal period, with an average age at onset between 4 and 6 years, and with the incidence of new-onset tic disorders decreasing in the teen years. New onset of tic symptoms in adulthood is exceedingly rare and is often associated with exposures to drugs (e.g., excessive cocaine use) or is a result of a central nervous system insult (e.g., postviral encephalitis). Although tic onset is uncommon in teenagers and adults, it is not uncommon for adolescents and adults to present for an initial diagnostic assessment and, when carefully evaluated, provide a history of milder symptoms dating back to childhood. New-onset abnormal movements suggestive of tics outside of the usual age range should result in evaluation for other movement disorders or for specific etiologies.

Tic symptoms cannot be attributable to the physiological effects of a substance or another medical condition (Criterion D). When there is strong evidence from the history, physical examination, and/or laboratory results to suggest a plausible, proximal, and probable cause for a tic disorder, a diagnosis of other specified tic disorder should be used.

Having previously met diagnostic criteria for Tourette's disorder negates a possible diagnosis of persistent (chronic) motor or vocal tic disorder (Criterion E). Similarly, a previous diagnosis of persistent (chronic) motor or vocal tic disorder negates a diagnosis of provisional tic disorder or other specified or unspecified tic disorder (Criterion E).

## Prevalence

Tics are common in childhood but transient in most cases. The estimated prevalence of Tourette's disorder ranges from 3 to 8 per 1,000 in school-age children. Males are more commonly affected than females, with the ratio varying from 2:1 to 4:1. A national survey in the United States estimated 3 per 1,000 for the prevalence of clinically identified cases. The frequency of identified cases was lower among African Americans and Hispanic Americans, which may be related to differences in access to care.

## Development and Course

Onset of tics is typically between ages 4 and 6 years. Peak severity occurs between ages 10 and 12 years, with a decline in severity during adolescence. Many adults with tic disorders experience diminished symptoms. A small percentage of individuals will have persistently severe or worsening symptoms in adulthood.

Tic symptoms manifest similarly in all age groups and across the lifespan. Tics wax and wane in severity and change in affected muscle groups and vocalizations over time. As children get older, they begin to report their tics being associated with a premonitory urge—a somatic sensation that precedes the tic—and a feeling of tension reduction following the expression of the tic. Tics associated with a premonitory urge may be experienced as not completely "involuntary" in that the urge and the tic can be resisted. An individual may also feel the need to perform a tic in a specific way or repeat it until he or she achieves the feeling that the tic has been done "just right."

The vulnerability toward developing co-occurring conditions changes as individuals pass through the age of risk for various co-occurring conditions. For example, prepubertal children with tic disorders are more likely to experience attention-deficit/hyperactivity disorder (ADHD), obsessive-compulsive disorder (OCD), and separation anxiety disorder than are teenagers and adults, who are more likely to experience the new onset of major depressive disorder, substance use disorder, or bipolar disorder.

## Risk and Prognostic Factors

**Temperamental.** Tics are worsened by anxiety, excitement, and exhaustion and are better during calm, focused activities. Individuals may have fewer tics when engaged in schoolwork or tasks at work than when relaxing at home after school or in the evening. Stressful/exciting events (e.g., taking a test, participating in exciting activities) often make tics worse.

**Environmental.** Observing a gesture or sound in another person may result in an individual with a tic disorder making a similar gesture or sound, which may be incorrectly perceived by others as purposeful. This can be a particular problem when the individual is interacting with authority figures (e.g., teachers, supervisors, police).

**Genetic and physiological.** Genetic and environmental factors influence tic symptom expression and severity. Important risk alleles for Tourette's disorder and rare genetic variants in families with tic disorders have been identified. Obstetrical complications, older paternal age, lower birth weight, and maternal smoking during pregnancy are associated with worse tic severity.

## Culture-Related Diagnostic Issues

Tic disorders do not appear to vary in clinical characteristics, course, or etiology by race, ethnicity, and culture. However, race, ethnicity, and culture may impact how tic disorders are perceived and managed in the family and community, as well as influencing patterns of help seeking, and choices of treatment.

## Gender-Related Diagnostic Issues

Males are more commonly affected than females, but there are no gender differences in the kinds of tics, age at onset, or course. Women with persistent tic disorders may be more likely to experience anxiety and depression.

## Functional Consequences of Tic Disorders

Many individuals with mild to moderate tic severity experience no distress or impairment in functioning and may even be unaware of their tics. Individuals with more severe symptoms generally have more impairment in daily living, but even individuals with moderate or even severe tic disorders may function well. The presence of a co-occurring condition, such as ADHD or OCD, can have greater impact on functioning. Less commonly, tics disrupt functioning in daily activities and result in social isolation, interpersonal conflict, peer victimization, inability to work or to go to school, and lower quality of life. The individual also may experience substantial psychological distress. Rare complications of Tourette's disorder include physical injury, such as eye injury (from hitting oneself in the face), and orthopedic and neurological injury (e.g., disc disease related to forceful head and neck movements).

# Differential Diagnosis

**Abnormal movements that may accompany other medical conditions and stereo-typic movement disorder.**   *Motor stereotypies* are defined as involuntary rhythmic, repetitive, predictable movements that appear purposeful but serve no obvious adaptive function or purpose and stop with distraction. Examples include repetitive hand waving/rotating, arm flapping, and finger wiggling. Motor stereotypies can be differentiated from tics based on the former's earlier age at onset (younger than 3 years), prolonged duration (seconds to minutes), constant repetitive fixed form and location, exacerbation when engrossed in activities, lack of a premonitory urge, and cessation with distraction (e.g., name called or touched). *Chorea* represents rapid, random, continual, abrupt, irregular, unpredictable, nonstereotyped actions that are usually bilateral and affect all parts of the body (i.e., face, trunk, and limbs). The timing, direction, and distribution of movements vary from moment to moment, and movements usually worsen during attempted voluntary action. *Dystonia* is the simultaneous sustained contracture of both agonist and antagonist muscles, resulting in a distorted posture or movement of parts of the body. Dystonic postures are often triggered by attempts at voluntary movements and are not seen during sleep.

**Substance-induced and paroxysmal dyskinesias.**   Paroxysmal dyskinesias usually occur as dystonic or choreoathetoid movements that are precipitated by voluntary movement or exertion and less commonly arise from normal background activity.

**Myoclonus.**   Myoclonus is characterized by a sudden unidirectional movement that is often nonrhythmic. It may be worsened by movement and occur during sleep. Myoclonus is differentiated from tics by its rapidity, lack of suppressibility, and absence of a premonitory urge.

**Obsessive-compulsive and related disorders.**   Differentiating obsessive-compulsive behaviors from tics may be difficult. Clues favoring an obsessive-compulsive behavior include a cognitive-based drive (e.g., fear of contamination) and the need to perform the action in a particular fashion a certain number of times, equally on both sides of the body, or until a "just right" feeling is achieved. Impulse-control problems and other repetitive behaviors, including persistent hair pulling, skin picking, and nail biting, appear more goal directed and complex than tics.

# Comorbidity

Many medical and psychiatric conditions have been described as co-occurring with tic disorders, with ADHD and obsessive-compulsive and related disorders being particularly common. The obsessive-compulsive symptoms observed in tic disorder tend to be characterized by more aggressive symmetry and order symptoms and poorer response to pharmacotherapy with selective serotonin reuptake inhibitors. Children with ADHD may demonstrate disruptive behavior, social immaturity, and learning difficulties that may interfere with academic progress and interpersonal relationships and lead to greater impairment than that caused by a tic disorder. Individuals with tic disorders can also have other movement disorders and other mental disorders, such as depressive, bipolar, or substance use disorders.

# Other Specified Tic Disorder

## 307.20 (F95.8)

This category applies to presentations in which symptoms characteristic of a tic disorder that cause clinically significant distress or impairment in social, occupational, or other important areas of functioning predominate but do not meet the full criteria for a tic disorder or any of the disorders in the neurodevelopmental disorders diagnostic class. The other specified tic disorder category is used in situations in which the clinician chooses to communicate the specific reason that the presentation does not meet the criteria for a tic disorder or any specific neurodevelopmental disorder. This is done by recording "other specified tic disorder" followed by the specific reason (e.g., "with onset after age 18 years").

# Unspecified Tic Disorder

## 307.20 (F95.9)

This category applies to presentations in which symptoms characteristic of a tic disorder that cause clinically significant distress or impairment in social, occupational, or other important areas of functioning predominate but do not meet the full criteria for a tic disorder or for any of the disorders in the neurodevelopmental disorders diagnostic class. The unspecified tic disorder category is used in situations in which the clinician chooses *not* to specify the reason that the criteria are not met for a tic disorder or for a specific neurodevelopmental disorder, and includes presentations in which there is insufficient information to make a more specific diagnosis.

# Other Neurodevelopmental Disorders

# Other Specified Neurodevelopmental Disorder

## 315.8 (F88)

This category applies to presentations in which symptoms characteristic of a neurodevelopmental disorder that cause impairment in social, occupational, or other important areas of functioning predominate but do not meet the full criteria for any of the disorders in the neurodevelopmental disorders diagnostic class. The other specified neurodevelopmental disorder category is used in situations in which the clinician chooses to communicate the specific reason that the presentation does not meet the criteria for any specific neurodevelopmental disorder. This is done by recording "other specified neurodevelopmental disorder" followed by the specific reason (e.g., "neurodevelopmental disorder associated with prenatal alcohol exposure").

An example of a presentation that can be specified using the "other specified" designation is the following:

**Neurodevelopmental disorder associated with prenatal alcohol exposure:** Neurodevelopmental disorder associated with prenatal alcohol exposure is characterized by a range of developmental disabilities following exposure to alcohol in utero.

# Unspecified Neurodevelopmental Disorder

## 315.9 (F89)

This category applies to presentations in which symptoms characteristic of a neurodevelopmental disorder that cause impairment in social, occupational, or other important areas of functioning predominate but do not meet the full criteria for any of the disorders in the neurodevelopmental disorders diagnostic class. The unspecified neurodevelopmental disorder category is used in situations in which the clinician chooses *not* to specify the reason that the criteria are not met for a specific neurodevelopmental disorder, and includes presentations in which there is insufficient information to make a more specific diagnosis (e.g., in emergency room settings).

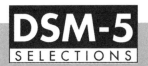

# Neurodevelopmental Disorders

## DSM-5® Guidebook

**Intellectual Disabilities**

|  | Intellectual Disability (Intellectual Developmental Disorder) |
|---|---|
| **317 (F70)** | Mild |
| **318.0 (F71)** | Moderate |
| **318.1 (F72)** | Severe |
| **318.2 (F73)** | Profound |
| **315.8 (F88)** | Global Developmental Delay |
| **319 (F79)** | Unspecified Intellectual Disability (Intellectual Developmental Disorder) |

**Communication Disorders**

| **315.32 (F80.2)** | Language Disorder |
|---|---|
| **315.39 (F80.0)** | Speech Sound Disorder |
| **315.35 (F80.81)** | Childhood-Onset Fluency Disorder (Stuttering) |
| **315.39 (F80.89)** | Social (Pragmatic) Communication Disorder |
| **307.9 (F80.9)** | Unspecified Communication Disorder |

**Autism Spectrum Disorder**

| **299.00 (F84.0)** | Autism Spectrum Disorder |
|---|---|

**Attention-Deficit/Hyperactivity Disorder**

|  | Attention-Deficit/Hyperactivity Disorder |
|---|---|
| **314.01 (F90.2)** | Combined Presentation |
| **314.00 (F90.0)** | Predominantly Inattentive Presentation |
| **314.01 (F90.1)** | Predominantly Hyperactive/Impulsive Presentation |
| **314.01 (F90.8)** | Other Specified Attention-Deficit/Hyperactivity Disorder |
| **314.01 (F90.9)** | Unspecified Attention-Deficit/Hyperactivity Disorder |

**Specific Learning Disorder**

|  | Specific Learning Disorder |
|---|---|
| **315.00 (F81.0)** | With Impairment in Reading |
| **315.2 (F81.81)** | With Impairment in Written Expression |
| **315.1 (F81.2)** | With Impairment in Mathematics |

**Motor Disorders**

| **315.4 (F82)** | Developmental Coordination Disorder |
|---|---|
| **307.3 (F98.4)** | Stereotypic Movement Disorder |

|  | Tic Disorders |
|---|---|
| **307.23 (F95.2)** | Tourette's Disorder |
| **307.22 (F95.1)** | Persistent (Chronic) Motor or Vocal Tic Disorder |
| **307.21 (F95.0)** | Provisional Tic Disorder |
| **307.20 (F95.8)** | Other Specified Tic Disorder |
| **307.20 (F95.9)** | Unspecified Tic Disorder |

**Other Neurodevelopmental Disorders**

| **315.8 (F88)** | Other Specified Neurodevelopmental Disorder |
|---|---|
| **315.9 (F89)** | Unspecified Neurodevelopmental Disorder |

This chapter is a reformulation of the DSM-IV chapter "Disorders Usually First Diagnosed in Infancy, Childhood, or Adolescence." The category was first included in DSM-III, which brought together intellectual disorders (under the rubric "mental retardation"), attention-deficit/hyperactivity disorder, conduct disorder, anxiety disorders of childhood, eating disorders, stereotypic movement disorders, and several other disorders. This represented an advance over the earlier editions, in which intellectual disorders were recognized but other childhood-onset disorders received little attention. In DSM-I, childhood disorders were subsumed within the categories mental deficiency, transient situational personality disturbances, adjustment reaction of infancy, adjustment reaction of adolescence, and adjustment reaction of childhood. The latter included such conditions as habit disturbances (i.e., nail biting, thumb sucking, enuresis, masturbation, tantrums, tics, habit spasms, somnambulism, overactivity, and phobias).

The term *mental retardation* was introduced in DSM-II (American Psychiatric Association 1968) to replace *mental deficiency*, and the category was expanded to include the variety of physical, infectious, and other causes of retardation. The category "behavior disorders of childhood and adolescence" was introduced to group together disorders "occurring in childhood and adolescence that are more stable, internalized, and resistant to treatment than *Transient situational disturbances* but less so than the *Psychoses, Neuroses,* and *Personality disorders*" (pp. 49–50). Included were hyperkinetic reaction, withdrawing reaction, overanxious reaction, runaway reaction, unsocialized aggressive reaction, and group delinquent reaction.

The authors of DSM-III brought together the intellectual, behavioral, emotional, physical, and developmental disorders that have their origins in infancy, childhood, or adolescence. An important contribution was the introduction of the *pervasive developmental disorders,* whose most prominent example was infantile autism and which had been recognized in one form or another for decades but never formally classified. Also new was the multiaxial system, in which mental retardation was coded on Axis II. As discussed in Chapter 2 [of the guidebook], "Use of DSM-5 and Major Changes From DSM-IV," the multiaxial system has been omitted from DSM-5. DSM-III-R and DSM-IV made further changes (e.g., creating a new chapter for eating disorders), but the category of early developing disorders remained largely unchanged.

Several major changes are highlighted in this chapter. First, its placement as the first class in DSM-5 is a reflection of the manual's metastructure and its emphasis on the developmental trajectory of disorders. Second, the term *mental retardation* has been replaced by *intellectual disability (intellectual developmental disorder)*. The revised diagnosis will capture those individuals formerly diagnosed with mental retardation, but there is no longer a reliance on IQ as the determinant for inclusion in the category. Instead, subtypes are used to classify the individual as having a mild, moderate, severe, or profound level of severity. The Neurodevelopmental Disorders Work Group considered the term *mental retardation* to be stigmatizing and no longer helpful. Further, the term *intellectual disability* reflects wording adopted into U.S. law in 2010 (Rosa's Law), and the term is used in professional journals and has been endorsed by some patient advocacy groups. The term *intellectual developmental disorder* is consistent with language proposed for ICD-11. Another concern expressed by the work group was the arbitrary reliance on IQ as the defining feature of intellectual disability, because it does not take into account the different domains of functioning (social, conceptual/intellectual, practical) that allow a more nuanced view of the person with an intellectual deficit.

Another major change in DSM-5 was the decision to create an omnibus category, autism spectrum disorder, that consolidates the DSM-IV categories autistic disorder, Rett's disorder, childhood disintegrative disorder, Asperger's disorder, and pervasive developmental disorder not otherwise specified. The change was prompted by research showing that the disorders were not as discrete and independent as once believed, and that clinicians had difficulty distinguishing them. All persons formerly included in each of these disorders should fit the new category, and its subtleties should be adequately captured by severity specifiers. This change has been criticized by clinicians, their patients, and the patients' parents. Parents expressed concern that the revised categories might leave their child unable to qualify for educational or other benefits, whereas individuals with Asperger's disorder who had developed a sense of identity felt disenfranchised.

Other changes to the class include moving oppositional defiant disorder and conduct disorder to the chapter "Disruptive, Impulse-Control, and Conduct Disorders." Elimination disorders (encopresis and enuresis) now have their own chapter, and the feeding disorders (pica, rumination disorder, and feeding disorder of infancy or early childhood) have been combined with the eating disorders for a more comprehensive chapter on disturbed eating behaviors. Separation anxiety disorder and selective mutism have been moved to the "Anxiety Disorders" chapter. Reactive attachment disorder has been moved to the "Trauma- and Stressor-Related Disorders" chapter because of its clear relationship with social neglect.

The communication disorders include language disorder, speech sound disorder, childhood-onset fluency disorder (stuttering), and social (pragmatic) communication disorder. The term *learning disorder* has been changed to *specific learning disorder,* and the previous types of learning disorders (reading disorder, mathematics disorder, and disorder of written expression) are no longer included. They are now presented as a single disorder with coded specifiers for deficits in reading, writing, and mathematics. Finally, other specified and unspecified attention-deficit/hyperactivity disorder diagnoses have been added (Table 1).

---

**TABLE 1.  DSM-5 neurodevelopmental disorders**

---

Intellectual disabilities
   Intellectual disability (intellectual developmental disorder)
   Global developmental delay
   Unspecified intellectual disability (intellectual developmental disorder)
Communication disorders
   Language disorder
   Speech sound disorder (previously phonological disorder)
   Childhood-onset fluency disorder (stuttering)
   Social (pragmatic) communication disorder
   Unspecified communication disorder
Autism spectrum disorder
Attention-deficit/hyperactivity disorder
   Attention-deficit/hyperactivity disorder
   Other specified attention-deficit/hyperactivity disorder
   Unspecified attention-deficit/hyperactivity disorder
Specific learning disorder
Motor disorders
   Developmental coordination disorder
   Stereotypic movement disorder
   Tourette's disorder
   Persistent (chronic) motor or vocal tic disorder
   Provisional tic disorder
   Other specified tic disorder
   Unspecified tic disorder
Other neurodevelopmental disorders
   Other specified neurodevelopmental disorder
   Unspecified neurodevelopmental disorder

---

# Intellectual Disabilities

## Intellectual Disability (Intellectual Developmental Disorder)

The essential features of intellectual disability (intellectual developmental disorder) are deficits in general mental abilities (Criterion A) and impairment in everyday adaptive functioning in comparison to the individual's age-, gender-, and socioculturally matched peers (Criterion B), with onset in the developmental period (Criterion C). Individuals with intellectual developmental disorder may also have difficulties in managing their behavior and emotions, in interpersonal relationships, and in maintaining motivation in the learning process.

The diagnosis is based on both clinical assessment and standardized testing of intelligence. *Intelligence* has been defined as a general mental ability that involves reasoning, problem solving, planning, thinking abstractly, comprehending complex ideas, judgment, academic learning, and learning from experience, as applied in academic learning and social understanding, as well as practical understanding and manipulation of objects. IQ is typically measured using standardized tests. With such tests, the category of intellectual disorder is considered to be about two standard deviations or more below the population mean, including a margin for measurement error (generally +5 points). On tests with a standard deviation of 15 and a mean of 100, this involves a score of 65–75. Clinical training and judgment are needed to interpret test results and assess intellectual performance. Factors other than intellectual developmental disorders, such as associated cultural background, native language, and communication disorders, may limit performance.

Intellectual developmental disorders are common (about 1%–2% of the general population), more so in boys than girls. These disorders almost certainly result from a final common pathway produced by a variety of factors that injure the brain and affect its normal development. Down syndrome is the most common chromosomal cause of mental retardation, whereas fragile X syndrome is probably the most common heritable form of intellectual disability. Inborn errors of metabolism (e.g., Tay-Sachs disease) account for a small percentage of cases. Other factors include maternal malnutrition or substance abuse; exposure to mutagens such as radiation; maternal illnesses such as diabetes, toxemia, or rubella; and maternal abuse and neglect. Perinatal and early postnatal factors also may contribute, such as traumatic deliveries that cause brain injury or malnutrition during infancy or early childhood.

Several important changes have been made to this category in DSM-5. The name was changed to *intellectual disability (intellectual developmental disorder)* from *mental retardation*, a term that is no longer used internationally or in U.S. federal legislation. The name *intellectual developmental disorder* was chosen to be consistent with DSM-5 as a classification of *disorders* and to harmonize this diagnosis with the proposed ICD-11. In DSM-5, IQ test scores and standard deviations from the mean on those tests, which were included in the diagnostic criteria for mental retardation in DSM-IV, have been moved to the body of the text and are not contained within the criteria. However, DSM-5 continues to specify that standardized psychological testing must be included in the assessment of persons with these disorders, consistent with the American Association on Intellectual and Developmental Disabilities (AAIDD) definition, but that psychological testing should accompany clinical assessment. With the elimination of the multiaxial classification in DSM-5, intellectual developmental disorder is no longer relegated to Axis II. Removing IQ ranges from the criteria means that IQ can no longer be used inappropriately to define a person's overall ability. Cognitive profiles are generally more useful than a single Full Scale IQ score for describing intellectual abilities, and clinical training and judgment are required for interpretation of test results.

Both AAIDD and DSM-5 define *intellectual functioning* as a general mental ability that involves reasoning, problem solving, planning, abstract thinking, comprehension of complex ideas, judgment, academic learning, and learning from experience. In DSM-5, the definition is applied to reasoning in three contexts: academic learning (conceptual domain), social understanding (social domain), and practical understanding (practical domain). A wide range of skills are contained within the three domains of adaptive behavior. The conceptual domain involves skills used to solve problems in language, reading, writing, math, reasoning, knowledge, and memory, among others. The social domain involves awareness of others' experiences, empathy, interpersonal communication skills, friendship abilities, social judgment, and self-regulation. The practical domain involves self-management across life settings, including personal care, job responsibilities, money management, recreation, managing one's behavior, and organizing school and work tasks.

With the inclusion of severity levels (mild, moderate, severe, profound) in DSM-5, the focus is on adaptive functioning rather than IQ. Adaptive functioning deficits are now required. *Adaptive functioning* refers to how well an individual copes with the common tasks of everyday life in three general domains (i.e., conceptual, social, and practical), and how well an individual meets the standards of personal independence and social responsibility expected for someone of a similar age, sociocultural background, and community setting in one or more aspects of daily life activities, such as communication, social participation, functioning at school or work, or personal independence at home or in community settings. For an individual with intellectual disability (intellectual developmental disorder), adaptive behavior limitations result in the need for ongoing support in school, work, or independent life.

## Diagnostic Criteria for Intellectual Disability (Intellectual Developmental Disorder)

Intellectual disability (intellectual developmental disorder) is a disorder with onset during the developmental period that includes both intellectual and adaptive functioning deficits in conceptual, social, and practical domains. The following three criteria must be met:

A. Deficits in intellectual functions, such as reasoning, problem solving, planning, abstract thinking, judgment, academic learning, and learning from experience, confirmed by both clinical assessment and individualized, standardized intelligence testing.

B. Deficits in adaptive functioning that result in failure to meet developmental and sociocultural standards for personal independence and social responsibility. Without ongoing support, the adaptive deficits limit functioning in one or more activities of daily life, such as communication, social participation, and independent living, across multiple environments, such as home, school, work, and community.

C. Onset of intellectual and adaptive deficits during the developmental period.

**Note:** The diagnostic term *intellectual disability* is the equivalent term for the ICD-11 diagnosis of *intellectual developmental disorders*. Although the term *intellectual disability* is used throughout this manual, both terms are used in the title to clarify relationships with other classification systems. Moreover, a federal statute in the United States (Public Law 111-256, Rosa's Law) replaces the term *mental retardation* with *intellectual disability,* and research journals use the term *intellectual disability.* Thus, *intellectual disability* is the term in common use by medical, educational, and other professions and by the lay public and advocacy groups.

*Specify* current severity (see Table 1 in DSM-5, pp. 34–36):
**317 (F70)   Mild**
**318.0 (F71) Moderate**
**318.1 (F72) Severe**
**318.2 (F73) Profound**

## Criteria A and B

Deficits in intellectual functions and impairment in adaptive functioning are both required in order for the diagnosis. For example, intellectual developmental disorder would not be recognized in an individual with an IQ score lower than 70 in the absence of significant deficits in adaptive functioning. The person must also have significant impairment in adaptive functioning (i.e., how well the person copes with the common tasks of everyday life and meets the standards of personal independence in social responsibility expected for someone of a similar age, sociocultural background, and community setting). Adaptive behavior reflects performance in academic, social, and practical settings in spite of intellectual ability, education, motivation, personality features, social and vocational opportunity, and coexisting medical conditions or mental disorders. When adaptive functioning is impaired, performance is limited and participation is restricted in one or more aspects of daily life activities, such as communication, social participation, and independent living, at home or in community settings.

## Criterion C

*Onset during the developmental period* refers to recognition and diagnosis before adolescence.

# Global Developmental Delay

Global developmental delay is a new diagnosis and allows the clinician to note cases in which evidence clearly indicates significant intellectual or general developmental delay or disability, but clinical severity level cannot be reliably assessed. The diagnosis is reserved for individuals under the age of 5 years.

| Global Developmental Delay | **315.8** (F88) |
|---|---|

This diagnosis is reserved for individuals *under* the age of 5 years when the clinical severity level cannot be reliably assessed during early childhood. This category is diagnosed when an individual fails to meet expected developmental milestones in several areas of intellectual functioning, and applies to individuals who are unable to undergo systematic assessments of intellectual functioning, including children who are too young to participate in standardized testing. This category requires reassessment after a period of time.

# Unspecified Intellectual Disability (Intellectual Developmental Disorder)

The diagnosis unspecified intellectual disability (intellectual developmental disorder) is used in persons over age 5 years who have significant intellectual or general developmental delay or disability and who cannot be reliably assessed.

## Unspecified Intellectual Disability (Intellectual Disability Disorder)                    **319** (F79)

This category is reserved for individuals *over* the age of 5 years when assessment of the degree of intellectual disability (intellectual developmental disorder) by means of locally available procedures is rendered difficult or impossible because of associated sensory or physical impairments, as in blindness or prelingual deafness; locomotor disability; or presence of severe problem behaviors or co-occurring mental disorder. This category should only be used in exceptional circumstances and requires reassessment after a period of time.

# Communication Disorders

The communication disorders are characterized by difficulties in language, speech, and communication. While not traditionally considered mental disorders, they can cause distress and impair functioning in important life domains and are important for purposes of differential diagnosis. The communication disorders include language disorder (which combines the DSM-IV categories expressive and mixed receptive-expressive language disorders), speech sound disorder (previously phonological disorder), and childhood-onset fluency disorder (previously stuttering). Social (pragmatic) communication disorder is a newly defined condition involving persistent difficulties in the social uses of verbal and nonverbal communication. DSM-IV *learning disorder* has been changed to *specific learning disorder,* and the previous types of learning disorders (reading disorder, mathematics disorder, and disorder of written expression) are no longer included. Instead, specifiers are used to describe the individual's impairment.

# Language Disorder

The essential feature of language disorder is a persistent disturbance in the acquisition and use of spoken language, written language, or sign language that is due to deficits in comprehension or production (Criterion A). Language abilities are substantially and quantifiably below those expected for age, significantly interfering with socialization, effective communication, academic achievement, or occupational performance (Criterion B). Regional variations in language (e.g., dialects) do not constitute a language disorder. Symptom onset is in the early developmental period (Criterion C). Other disorders (e.g., intellectual disability [intellectual developmental disorder], hearing impairment, motor dysfunction) must be ruled out as a cause of the language difficulties (Criterion D).

---

## Diagnostic Criteria for Language Disorder       **315.32 (F80.2)**

A. Persistent difficulties in the acquisition and use of language across modalities (i.e., spoken, written, sign language, or other) due to deficits in comprehension or production that include the following:
   1. Reduced vocabulary (word knowledge and use).
   2. Limited sentence structure (ability to put words and word endings together to form sentences based on the rules of grammar and morphology).
   3. Impairments in discourse (ability to use vocabulary and connect sentences to explain or describe a topic or series of events or have a conversation).
B. Language abilities are substantially and quantifiably below those expected for age, resulting in functional limitations in effective communication, social participation, academic achievement, or occupational performance, individually or in any combination.
C. Onset of symptoms is in the early developmental period.
D. The difficulties are not attributable to hearing or other sensory impairment, motor dysfunction, or another medical or neurological condition and are not better explained by intellectual disability (intellectual developmental disorder) or global developmental delay.

---

# Speech Sound Disorder

Speech sound disorder is characterized by persistent difficulties in speech production that are developmentally inappropriate and involve articulation, fluency, and voice production in its various aspects. This disorder often coexists with language disorder, intellectual disability (intellectual developmental disorder), and neurological conditions such as Landau-Kleffner syndrome.

Diagnostic Criteria for Speech Sound Disorder          **315.39** (F80.0)

A. Persistent difficulty with speech sound production that interferes with speech intelligibility or prevents verbal communication of messages.
B. The disturbance causes limitations in effective communication that interfere with social participation, academic achievement, or occupational performance, individually or in any combination.
C. Onset of symptoms is in the early developmental period.
D. The difficulties are not attributable to congenital or acquired conditions, such as cerebral palsy, cleft palate, deafness or hearing loss, traumatic brain injury, or other medical or neurological conditions.

# Childhood-Onset Fluency Disorder (Stuttering)

Childhood-onset fluency disorder (stuttering) is characterized by a disturbance in the normal fluency and time patterning of speech that is inappropriate for age. The disturbance can manifest as frequent repetitions or prolongations of sounds or syllables or other types of speech dysfluencies, such as sound and syllable repetitions, broken words (e.g., pauses within a word), audible or silent blocking (e.g., filled or unfilled pauses in speech), or circumlocutions (e.g., word substitutions to avoid problematic words). The disturbance interferes with academic or occupational achievement or with social communication. Stuttering can also cause humiliation and embarrassment and lead individuals to avoid situations that may be associated with speech, such as using a telephone. The disorder usually occurs by age 6 years, although most recover from the dysfluency. Stress and anxiety can exacerbate the disorder.

Diagnostic Criteria for Childhood-Onset
Fluency Disorder (Stuttering)                          **315.35** (F80.81)

A. Disturbances in the normal fluency and time patterning of speech that are inappropriate for the individual's age and language skills, persist over time, and are characterized by frequent and marked occurrences of one (or more) of the following:
   1. Sound and syllable repetitions.
   2. Sound prolongations of consonants as well as vowels.
   3. Broken words (e.g., pauses within a word).
   4. Audible or silent blocking (filled or unfilled pauses in speech).
   5. Circumlocutions (word substitutions to avoid problematic words).
   6. Words produced with an excess of physical tension.
   7. Monosyllabic whole-word repetitions (e.g., "I-I-I-I see him").
B. The disturbance causes anxiety about speaking or limitations in effective communication, social participation, or academic or occupational performance, individually or in any combination.

C. The onset of symptoms is in the early developmental period. (**Note:** Later-onset cases are diagnosed as 307.0 [F98.5] adult-onset fluency disorder.)

D. The disturbance is not attributable to a speech-motor or sensory deficit, dysfluency associated with neurological insult (e.g., stroke, tumor, trauma), or another medical condition and is not better explained by another mental disorder.

# Social (Pragmatic) Communication Disorder

Social (pragmatic) communication disorder is new to DSM-5. This is a disorder of children who have difficulty with the pragmatic aspects of social communication, including comprehension, formulation, and discourse comprehension, affecting idiomatic and nonliteral language inferences in narrative texts and conversation (Bishop 2000). This disorder is unexpected given a child's relatively intact vocabulary and sentence abilities. Research suggests that such children exhibit socially inappropriate behavior but do not have autism spectrum disorder (Bishop and Norbury 2002). Thus, the pragmatic difficulties they experience constitute a fundamentally different form of language impairment. Children with this condition display common difficulties in social communication but not repetitive behaviors or restricted interests consistent with autism spectrum disorder. Autism spectrum disorder needs to be ruled out, as do attention-deficit/hyperactivity disorder, social anxiety disorder, and intellectual disability (intellectual developmental disorder).

## Diagnostic Criteria for Social (Pragmatic) Communication Disorder **315.39** (F80.89)

A. Persistent difficulties in the social use of verbal and nonverbal communication as manifested by all of the following:

1. Deficits in using communication for social purposes, such as greeting and sharing information, in a manner that is appropriate for the social context.

2. Impairment of the ability to change communication to match context or the needs of the listener, such as speaking differently in a classroom than on a playground, talking differently to a child than to an adult, and avoiding use of overly formal language.

3. Difficulties following rules for conversation and storytelling, such as taking turns in conversation, rephrasing when misunderstood, and knowing how to use verbal and nonverbal signals to regulate interaction.

4. Difficulties understanding what is not explicitly stated (e.g., making inferences) and nonliteral or ambiguous meanings of language (e.g., idioms, humor, metaphors, multiple meanings that depend on the context for interpretation).

B. The deficits result in functional limitations in effective communication, social participation, social relationships, academic achievement, or occupational performance, individually or in combination.

C. The onset of the symptoms is in the early developmental period (but deficits may not become fully manifest until social communication demands exceed limited capacities).

D. The symptoms are not attributable to another medical or neurological condition or to low abilities in the domains of word structure and grammar, and are not better explained by autism spectrum disorder, intellectual disability (intellectual developmental disorder), global developmental delay, or another mental disorder.

# Unspecified Communication Disorder

| Unspecified Communication Disorder | **307.9** (F80.9) |
|---|---|

This category applies to presentations in which symptoms characteristic of communication disorder that cause clinically significant distress or impairment in social, occupational, or other important areas of functioning predominate but do not meet the full criteria for communication disorder or for any of the disorders in the neurodevelopmental disorders diagnostic class. The unspecified communication disorder category is used in situations in which the clinician chooses *not* to specify the reason that the criteria are not met for communication disorder or for a specific neurodevelopmental disorder, and includes presentations in which there is insufficient information to make a more specific diagnosis.

# Autism Spectrum Disorder

## Autism Spectrum Disorder

Autism was described by Leo Kanner (1948) as a syndrome of social communication deficits combined with repetitive and stereotyped behaviors and as having an onset in early childhood. In DSM-III, the disorder was called "infantile autism" and was listed as one of several pervasive developmental disorders. In DSM-III-R and DSM-IV, other related disorders were included in the category, including Rett's disorder, childhood disintegrative disorder, Asperger's disorder, and pervasive developmental disorder not otherwise specified. DSM-5 now replaces all of these diagnoses with a single diagnosis, autism spectrum disorder. Autism spectrum disorder is considered a neurodevelopmental disorder. Although present from infancy or early childhood, the disorder may not be detected until later because of minimal social demands and support from parents or caregivers in early years.

For DSM-5, the diagnosis has been reconceptualized as a "spectrum" that includes all of the various disorders previously distinguished in DSM-IV. The essential features of autism spectrum disorder are persistent deficits in reciprocal social communication, in nonverbal communicative behaviors used for social interaction, and in developing, managing, and understanding relationships (Criterion A) and restricted, repetitive patterns of behavior, interests, or activities (Criterion B). Distinctions among the pervasive developmental disorders were inconsistent over time, variable across sites, and often associated with severity, language level, or intelligence rather than features of the disorder. The Neurodevelopmental Disorders Work Group considered various options and concluded that because autism is defined by a common set of behaviors, it is best represented as a single diagnostic category adapted to the individual's clinical presentation by inclusion of clinical specifiers (e.g., severity, intellectual impairment, language impairment) and associated features (e.g., known genetic disorders, epilepsy, intellectual disability). For example, an individual formerly diagnosed with Asperger's disorder can now be diagnosed with autism spectrum disorder, without intellectual impairment and without accompanying structural language impairment.

The work group made other changes to the category. The three domains in DSM-IV (social interaction, communication, repetitive/stereotyped behaviors) have become two: 1) social-communication and social-interactive deficits and 2) restricted, repetitive behaviors, interests, and activities. Research shows that deficits in communication and social behaviors are inseparable and best considered as a single set of symptoms with contextual and environmental specificities. Also, delays in language acquisition are neither unique nor universal, and are more accurately considered as a factor that influences the clinical symptoms of autism spectrum disorder rather than as a feature that defines the diagnosis. Requiring that both criteria be met improves specificity of diagnosis without impairing sensitivity.

---

## Diagnostic Criteria for Autism Spectrum Disorder    **299.00** (F84.0)

A. Persistent deficits in social communication and social interaction across multiple contexts, as manifested by the following, currently or by history (examples are illustrative, not exhaustive; see DSM-5 text):

1. Deficits in social-emotional reciprocity, ranging, for example, from abnormal social approach and failure of normal back-and-forth conversation; to reduced sharing of interests, emotions, or affect; to failure to initiate or respond to social interactions.

2. Deficits in nonverbal communicative behaviors used for social interaction, ranging, for example, from poorly integrated verbal and nonverbal communication; to abnormalities in eye contact and body language or deficits in understanding and use of gestures; to a total lack of facial expressions and nonverbal communication.

3. Deficits in developing, maintaining, and understanding relationships, ranging, for example, from difficulties adjusting behavior to suit various social contexts; to difficulties in sharing imaginative play or in making friends; to absence of interest in peers.

*Specify* current severity:

**Severity is based on social communication impairments and restricted, repetitive patterns of behavior** (see Table 2 in DSM-5, p. 52).

B. Restricted, repetitive patterns of behavior, interests, or activities, as manifested by at least two of the following, currently or by history (examples are illustrative, not exhaustive; see DSM-5 text):

1. Stereotyped or repetitive motor movements, use of objects, or speech (e.g., simple motor stereotypies, lining up toys or flipping objects, echolalia, idiosyncratic phrases).

2. Insistence on sameness, inflexible adherence to routines, or ritualized patterns of verbal or nonverbal behavior (e.g., extreme distress at small changes, difficulties with transitions, rigid thinking patterns, greeting rituals, need to take same route or eat same food every day).

3. Highly restricted, fixated interests that are abnormal in intensity or focus (e.g., strong attachment to or preoccupation with unusual objects, excessively circumscribed or perseverative interests).

4. Hyper- or hyporeactivity to sensory input or unusual interest in sensory aspects of the environment (e.g., apparent indifference to pain/temperature, adverse response to specific sounds or textures, excessive smelling or touching of objects, visual fascination with lights or movement).

*Specify* current severity:

**Severity is based on social communication impairments and restricted, repetitive patterns of behavior** (see Table 2 in DSM-5, p. 52).

C. Symptoms must be present in the early developmental period (but may not become fully manifest until social demands exceed limited capacities, or may be masked by learned strategies in later life).

D. Symptoms cause clinically significant impairment in social, occupational, or other important areas of current functioning.

E. These disturbances are not better explained by intellectual disability (intellectual developmental disorder) or global developmental delay. Intellectual disability and autism spectrum disorder frequently co-occur; to make comorbid diagnoses of autism spectrum disorder and intellectual disability, social communication should be below that expected for general developmental level.

**Note:** Individuals with a well-established DSM-IV diagnosis of autistic disorder, Asperger's disorder, or pervasive developmental disorder not otherwise specified should be given the diagnosis of autism spectrum disorder. Individuals who have marked deficits in social communication, but whose symptoms do not otherwise meet criteria for autism spectrum disorder, should be evaluated for social (pragmatic) communication disorder.

*Specify* if:

**With or without accompanying intellectual impairment**

**With or without accompanying language impairment**

**Associated with a known medical or genetic condition or environmental factor** (**Coding note:** Use additional code to identify the associated medical or genetic condition.)

**Associated with another neurodevelopmental, mental, or behavioral disorder** (**Coding note:** Use additional code[s] to identify the associated neurodevelopmental, mental, or behavioral disorder[s].)

**With catatonia** (refer to the criteria for catatonia associated with another mental disorder, DSM-5, pp. 119–120, for definition) (**Coding note:** Use additional code 293.89 [F06.1] catatonia associated with autism spectrum disorder to indicate the presence of the comorbid catatonia.)

## Criterion A

The essential feature of autism spectrum disorder is persistent impairment in reciprocal social communication and social interaction across multiple contexts. This symptom is pervasive and sustained. Manifestations depend in part on age, intellectual level, and language ability, as well as on individual differences in personality and other factors, such as treatment history and current support. For many with this disorder, language will be affected (e.g., speech may be absent or its onset delayed). Communication may be impaired even when formal skills, including vocabulary and grammar, are intact. Deficits in social-emotional reciprocity are clearly evident, and young children with the disorder may show little or no initiation of social interaction and no sharing of emotions. An early feature is poor or absent eye contact.

## Criterion B

This criterion requires the child to have restricted, repetitive patterns of behavior, interests, or activities. For example, the child may prefer rigid routines and insist that things be done in the same way. The child may have a narrow and intense focus on particular topics, such as train schedules. The child may exhibit stereotyped or repetitive behaviors, such as hand flapping or finger flicking. Excessive adherence to routines and restricted patterns of behavior may be manifested as resistance to change or ritualized patterns of verbal or nonverbal behavior, such as repetitive questioning. Highly restricted, fixated interests tend to be abnormal in intensity and/or focus (e.g., preoccupation with vacuum cleaners). Interests and routines may relate to high or low levels of reactivity to sensory input, as shown by extreme responses to specific sounds or textures, excessive smelling or touching of objects, fascination with lights or spinning objects, and sometimes apparent indifference to pain, heat, or cold.

## Criteria C, D, and E

Symptoms begin early in life and limit or cause impairments in social, occupational, or other critical areas of functioning. The stage at which functional impairment becomes apparent varies by individual and his or her environment. Core diagnostic features are evident in the developmental period, but intervention, compensation, and current supports may mask difficulties at later stages of the disorder.

Autism spectrum disorder needs to be differentiated from intellectual disability (intellectual developmental disorder) and global developmental delay, because the latter conditions can be associated with communication difficulties. The distinction may be particularly difficult in young children. The determination may rest on whether the communication and interaction are significantly impaired relative to the developmental level of the individual's nonverbal skills, in which case the diagnosis of autism spectrum disorder is likely.

Children with an autism spectrum disorder may have relatively obvious problems early in life. Within the first 3–6 months, parents may note that their child does not develop a normal pattern of smiling or responding to cuddling. The first clear sign of abnormality is usually in the area of language. As the child grows older, he or she does not progress through developmental milestones, such as learning to say words and speak sentences, and seems aloof, withdrawn, and detached. Instead of developing patterns of relating warmly to his or her parents, the child may instead engage in self-stimulating behavior, such as rocking or head banging. Eventually, it becomes clear that something is severely wrong, and the features of the disorder continue to become more apparent over time as these children fail to develop normal verbal and interpersonal communication.

In young children, lack of social and communication abilities may hamper learning, especially that associated with social interactions. In the home, insistence on routines and aversion to change, as well as sensory sensitivities, may interfere with eating and sleeping and make routine care (e.g., haircuts, dental appointments) extremely difficult. In adulthood, rigidity and difficulty with novelty may limit independence even in highly intelligent people with autism spectrum disorder.

# Attention-Deficit/Hyperactivity Disorder

## Attention-Deficit/Hyperactivity Disorder

Attention-deficit/hyperactivity disorder (ADHD) was first acknowledged in DSM-II as a hyperkinetic reaction of childhood (or adolescence), characterized by overactivity, restlessness, distractibility, and short attention span. DSM-III provided operational diagnostic criteria and emphasized deficits in attention, impulsivity, and hyperactivity, but included a category for those without hyperactivity. In DSM-IV, the criteria were revised to focus on two broad groups of symptoms: 1) difficulty focusing and maintaining attention and 2) hyperactivity and impulsivity. The criteria required that at least 12 of 18 symptoms (6 from the domain of attention and 6 from the domain of hyperactivity-impulsivity) be present for at least 6 months, with onset before age 7 years. Subtypes could be used to specify whether the presentation was predominantly inattentive, predominantly hyperactive-impulsive, or mixed. Several changes have been made to the diagnosis in DSM-5. First, age at onset has been changed from onset of impairing symptoms by age 7 to onset of symptoms by age 12. Research has shown that estimates of onset by age 7 years are unreliable and that few clinical differences exist between children identified as having onset by age 7 versus those with later onset in terms of course, severity, outcome, or treatment response (Applegate et al. 1997). Subtypes have been replaced with presentation specifiers that map directly to the prior subtypes. Examples used in the criterion items have been changed to accommodate a life span relevance of each symptom and to improve clarity (Matte et al. 2012). Symptom threshold for adults age 17 years or older was reduced to five (from six for those younger than 17 years) both for inattention and for hyperactivity and impulsivity. The change was prompted by research showing that individuals tend to have fewer symptoms of ADHD in adulthood than in childhood. Finally, in response to data showing that ADHD and autism spectrum disorder can coexist, a comorbid diagnosis with autism spectrum disorder is now allowed. This change brings the ADHD criteria into harmony with the revised criteria for autism spectrum disorder.

## Diagnostic Criteria for Attention-Deficit/Hyperactivity Disorder

A. A persistent pattern of inattention and/or hyperactivity-impulsivity that interferes with functioning or development, as characterized by (1) and/or (2):

1. **Inattention:** Six (or more) of the following symptoms have persisted for at least 6 months to a degree that is inconsistent with developmental level and that negatively impacts directly on social and academic/occupational activities:
   **Note:** The symptoms are not solely a manifestation of oppositional behavior, defiance, hostility, or failure to understand tasks or instructions. For older adolescents and adults (age 17 and older), at least five symptoms are required.

   a. Often fails to give close attention to details or makes careless mistakes in schoolwork, at work, or during other activities (e.g., overlooks or misses details, work is inaccurate).
   b. Often has difficulty sustaining attention in tasks or play activities (e.g., has difficulty remaining focused during lectures, conversations, or lengthy reading).
   c. Often does not seem to listen when spoken to directly (e.g., mind seems elsewhere, even in the absence of any obvious distraction).
   d. Often does not follow through on instructions and fails to finish schoolwork, chores, or duties in the workplace (e.g., starts tasks but quickly loses focus and is easily sidetracked).
   e. Often has difficulty organizing tasks and activities (e.g., difficulty managing sequential tasks; difficulty keeping materials and belongings in order; messy, disorganized work; has poor time management; fails to meet deadlines).
   f. Often avoids, dislikes, or is reluctant to engage in tasks that require sustained mental effort (e.g., schoolwork or homework; for older adolescents and adults, preparing reports, completing forms, reviewing lengthy papers).
   g. Often loses things necessary for tasks or activities (e.g., school materials, pencils, books, tools, wallets, keys, paperwork, eyeglasses, mobile telephones).
   h. Is often easily distracted by extraneous stimuli (for older adolescents and adults, may include unrelated thoughts).
   i. Is often forgetful in daily activities (e.g., doing chores, running errands; for older adolescents and adults, returning calls, paying bills, keeping appointments).

2. **Hyperactivity and impulsivity:** Six (or more) of the following symptoms have persisted for at least 6 months to a degree that is inconsistent with developmental level and that negatively impacts directly on social and academic/occupational activities:

**Note:** The symptoms are not solely a manifestation of oppositional behavior, defiance, hostility, or a failure to understand tasks or instructions. For older adolescents and adults (age 17 and older), at least five symptoms are required.

   a. Often fidgets with or taps hands or feet or squirms in seat.
   b. Often leaves seat in situations when remaining seated is expected (e.g., leaves his or her place in the classroom, in the office or other workplace, or in other situations that require remaining in place).
   c. Often runs about or climbs in situations where it is inappropriate. (**Note:** In adolescents or adults, may be limited to feeling restless.)
   d. Often unable to play or engage in leisure activities quietly.
   e. Is often "on the go," acting as if "driven by a motor" (e.g., is unable to be or uncomfortable being still for extended time, as in restaurants, meetings; may be experienced by others as being restless or difficult to keep up with).
   f. Often talks excessively.
   g. Often blurts out an answer before a question has been completed (e.g., completes people's sentences; cannot wait for turn in conversation).
   h. Often has difficulty waiting his or her turn (e.g., while waiting in line).
   i. Often interrupts or intrudes on others (e.g., butts into conversations, games, or activities; may start using other people's things without asking or receiving permission; for adolescents and adults, may intrude into or take over what others are doing).

B. Several inattentive or hyperactive-impulsive symptoms were present prior to age 12 years.
C. Several inattentive or hyperactive-impulsive symptoms are present in two or more settings (e.g., at home, school, or work; with friends or relatives; in other activities).
D. There is clear evidence that the symptoms interfere with, or reduce the quality of, social, academic, or occupational functioning.
E. The symptoms do not occur exclusively during the course of schizophrenia or another psychotic disorder and are not better explained by another mental disorder (e.g., mood disorder, anxiety disorder, dissociative disorder, personality disorder, substance intoxication or withdrawal).

*Specify* whether:

**314.01 (F90.2) Combined presentation:** If both Criterion A1 (inattention) and Criterion A2 (hyperactivity-impulsivity) are met for the past 6 months.

**314.00 (F90.0) Predominantly inattentive presentation:** If Criterion A1 (inattention) is met but Criterion A2 (hyperactivity-impulsivity) is not met for the past 6 months.

**314.01 (F90.1) Predominantly hyperactive/impulsive presentation:** If Criterion A2 (hyperactivity-impulsivity) is met and Criterion A1 (inattention) is not met for the past 6 months.

*Specify* if:

**In partial remission:** When full criteria were previously met, fewer than the full criteria have been met for the past 6 months, and the symptoms still result in impairment in social, academic, or occupational functioning.

*Specify* current severity:

**Mild:** Few, if any, symptoms in excess of those required to make the diagnosis are present, and symptoms result in no more than minor impairments in social or occupational functioning.

**Moderate:** Symptoms or functional impairment between "mild" and "severe" are present.

**Severe:** Many symptoms in excess of those required to make the diagnosis, or several symptoms that are particularly severe, are present, or the symptoms result in marked impairment in social or occupational functioning.

## Criterion A

The essential feature of ADHD is a persistent pattern of inattention (Criterion A1) and/or hyperactivity-impulsivity (Criterion A2) sufficiently severe that it interferes with functioning or development. *Inattention* refers to problems with the following: staying on task, being persistent, focusing, being organized, planning, and following through. *Hyperactivity* is manifested as excessive motor activity, such as running about or climbing, or excessive fidgeting, tapping, or squirming, in situations where it is not appropriate. Hyperactivity may not be continuous, but overactivity may occur very frequently.

## Criterion B

This item requires that several symptoms of ADHD have an onset before age 12 years because it is difficult to reliably establish precise childhood onset retrospectively (Kieling et al. 2010). For adolescents or young adults, a longitudinal perspective should indicate that the condition had its roots during childhood and is not of recent onset.

## Criterion C

This item requires that several symptoms of ADHD appear in two or more settings. Although potentially costly and time consuming, and while not a requirement for diagnosis, the text recommends consulting informants (e.g., parents, teachers, employers) who have seen the individual across various settings. For children, teacher rating scales can provide valuable and adjunctive information as to expectations for normative patterns of behavior.

## Criterion D

In children, ADHD can impair school performance. In adults, worse occupational performance and attendance, higher probability of unemployment, interpersonal conflict, and reduced self-esteem are common. Children with ADHD are about twice as likely as children without a disorder to experience an injury requiring medical attention, presumably due to their impulsivity and inattention. Inadequate self-application to tasks that require sustained effort is often interpreted by others as laziness, a poor sense of responsibility, and oppositional behavior. Family relationships are often characterized by resentment and antagonism, especially because variability in the person's symptomatic status often leads others to believe that the troublesome behavior is willful.

## Criterion E

Other mental disorders need to be ruled out as a cause for the symptoms. ADHD shares symptoms of inattention with both anxiety disorders and major depression. Individuals with ADHD are inattentive due to daydreaming or their attraction to external stimuli or new activities. ADHD should be readily distinguished from the inattention due to worry, rumination, and internal stimuli seen with anxiety disorders or major depression. Young people with bipolar disorder may have increased activity, but the activity is episodic, varying with mood and goal-directed behavior. ADHD should not be confused with mania. Disruptive mood dysregulation disorder is characterized by consistent moodiness, irritability, and intolerance of frustration, but impulsivity and disorganized attention are not part of the condition.

In some adults, distinguishing ADHD from various personality disorders (e.g., antisocial, borderline, narcissistic) may be difficult. These disorders tend to share the features of disorganization, social intrusiveness, emotional dysregulation, and cognitive dysregulation. However, ADHD is not characterized by fears of abandonment, self-injury, extreme ambivalence, or other features of severe personality disorders. Lastly, ADHD is not diagnosed if the symptoms of inattention and hyperactivity occur exclusively during the course of a psychotic disorder.

# Other Specified Attention-Deficit/Hyperactivity Disorder and Unspecified Attention-Deficit/Hyperactivity Disorder

Other specified ADHD and unspecified ADHD are residual categories for those presentations of ADHD that do not fit within the more specific diagnostic category.

## Other Specified Attention-Deficit/Hyperactivity Disorder                                         **314.01** (F90.8)

This category applies to presentations in which symptoms characteristic of attention-deficit/hyperactivity disorder that cause clinically significant distress or impairment in social, occupational or other important areas of functioning predominate but do not meet the full criteria for attention-deficit/hyperactivity disorder or any of the disorders in the neurodevelopmental disorders diagnostic class. The other specified attention-deficit/hyperactivity disorder category is used in situations in which the clinician chooses to communicate the specific reason that the presentation does not meet the criteria for attention-deficit/hyperactivity disorder or any specific neurodevelopmental disorder. This is done by recording "other specified attention-deficit/hyperactivity disorder" followed by the specific reason (e.g., "with insufficient inattention symptoms").

## Unspecified Attention-Deficit/Hyperactivity Disorder   **314.01** (F90.9)

This category applies to presentations in which symptoms characteristic of attention-deficit/hyperactivity disorder that cause clinically significant distress or impairment in social, occupational, or other important areas of functioning predominate but do not meet the full criteria for attention-deficit/hyperactivity disorder or any of the disorders in the neurodevelopmental disorders diagnostic class. The unspecified attention-deficit/hyperactivity disorder category is used in situations in which the clinician chooses *not* to specify the reason that the criteria are not met for attention-deficit/hyperactivity disorder or for a specific neurodevelopmental disorder, and includes presentations in which there is insufficient information to make a more specific diagnosis.

# Specific Learning Disorder

## Specific Learning Disorder

Specific learning disorder is characterized by persistent difficulties in learning and using academic skills, with onset during the developmental period. Specific learning disorder is a clinical diagnosis based on a synthesis of the person's medical, developmental, educational, and family history; the history of the learning difficulty and its manifestation; the impact on academic, occupational, or social functioning; observations as the person reads or solves age- or grade-level material; school reports; and scores from individual standardized educational or neuropsychological testing. This diagnosis replaces reading disorder, mathematics disorder, and disorder of written expression. Instead, these disorders are now included in a single diagnosis with coded specifiers for impairments in reading, written expression, and mathematics. The reason for the change was widespread concern among clinicians and researchers that DSM-IV's three independent learning disorders lacked validity. This change is particularly important given that most children with a specific learning disorder manifest deficits in more than one area. With the reclassification of these conditions as a single disorder, separate specifiers can be used to code the specific deficits present in each of the three areas as well as current severity. Specific types of reading disorders are widely described as *dyslexia*, while specific types of mathematics deficits are described as *dyscalculia*.

The essential feature is a persistent problem in learning or using academic skills as quickly or as accurately as peers during the developmental period (Criterion A). Thus, the individual's academic skills are well below the average range for his or her age, gender-based peers, and cultural group (Criterion B). The clinical expression of the specific learning difficulties occurs during the school-age years, and therefore these difficulties may not be apparent until demands on the affected skills exceed the individual's abilities (Criterion C). The learning difficulties cannot be accounted for by intellectual difficulties, uncorrected visual or auditory problems, psychosocial adversity, poor proficiency in the language of academic instruction, or inadequate educational instruction (Criterion D).

## Diagnostic Criteria for Specific Learning Disorder

A. Difficulties learning and using academic skills, as indicated by the presence of at least one of the following symptoms that have persisted for at least 6 months, despite the provision of interventions that target those difficulties:

1. Inaccurate or slow and effortful word reading (e.g., reads single words aloud incorrectly or slowly and hesitantly, frequently guesses words, has difficulty sounding out words).
2. Difficulty understanding the meaning of what is read (e.g., may read text accurately but not understand the sequence, relationships, inferences, or deeper meanings of what is read).
3. Difficulties with spelling (e.g., may add, omit, or substitute vowels or consonants).
4. Difficulties with written expression (e.g., makes multiple grammatical or punctuation errors within sentences; employs poor paragraph organization; written expression of ideas lacks clarity).
5. Difficulties mastering number sense, number facts, or calculation (e.g., has poor understanding of numbers, their magnitude, and relationships; counts on fingers to add single-digit numbers instead of recalling the math fact as peers do; gets lost in the midst of arithmetic computation and may switch procedures).
6. Difficulties with mathematical reasoning (e.g., has severe difficulty applying mathematical concepts, facts, or procedures to solve quantitative problems).

B. The affected academic skills are substantially and quantifiably below those expected for the individual's chronological age, and cause significant interference with academic or occupational performance, or with activities of daily living, as confirmed by individually administered standardized achievement measures and comprehensive clinical assessment. For individuals age 17 years and older, a documented history of impairing learning difficulties may be substituted for the standardized assessment.

C. The learning difficulties begin during school-age years but may not become fully manifest until the demands for those affected academic skills exceed the individual's limited capacities (e.g., as in timed tests, reading or writing lengthy complex reports for a tight deadline, excessively heavy academic loads).

D. The learning difficulties are not better accounted for by intellectual disabilities, uncorrected visual or auditory acuity, other mental or neurological disorders, psychosocial adversity, lack of proficiency in the language of academic instruction, or inadequate educational instruction.

**Note:** The four diagnostic criteria are to be met based on a clinical synthesis of the individual's history (developmental, medical, family, educational), school reports, and psychoeducational assessment.

**Coding note:** Specify all academic domains and subskills that are impaired. When more than one domain is impaired, each one should be coded individually according to the following specifiers.

*Specify* if:

**315.00 (F81.0) With impairment in reading:**

Word reading accuracy

Reading rate or fluency

Reading comprehension

**Note:** *Dyslexia* is an alternative term used to refer to a pattern of learning difficulties characterized by problems with accurate or fluent word recognition, poor decoding, and poor spelling abilities. If dyslexia is used to specify this particular pattern of difficulties, it is important also to specify any additional difficulties that are present, such as difficulties with reading comprehension or math reasoning.

**315.2 (F81.81) With impairment in written expression:**

Spelling accuracy

Grammar and punctuation accuracy

Clarity or organization of written expression

**315.1 (F81.2) With impairment in mathematics:**

Number sense

Memorization of arithmetic facts

Accurate or fluent calculation

Accurate math reasoning

**Note:** *Dyscalculia* is an alternative term used to refer to a pattern of difficulties characterized by problems processing numerical information, learning arithmetic facts, and performing accurate or fluent calculations. If dyscalculia is used to specify this particular pattern of mathematic difficulties, it is important also to specify any additional difficulties that are present, such as difficulties with math reasoning or word reasoning accuracy.

*Specify* current severity:

**Mild:** Some difficulties learning skills in one or two academic domains, but of mild enough severity that the individual may be able to compensate or function well when provided with appropriate accommodations or support services, especially during the school years.

**Moderate:** Marked difficulties learning skills in one or more academic domains, so that the individual is unlikely to become proficient without some intervals of intensive and specialized teaching during the school years. Some accommodations or supportive services at least part of the day at school, in the workplace, or at home may be needed to complete activities accurately and efficiently.

**Severe:** Severe difficulties learning skills, affecting several academic domains, so that the individual is unlikely to learn those skills without ongoing intensive individualized and specialized teaching for most of the school years. Even with an array of appropriate accommodations or services at home, at school, or in the workplace, the individual may not be able to complete all activities efficiently.

# Motor Disorders

## Developmental Coordination Disorder

The essential feature of developmental coordination disorder is a marked impairment in the developmental acquisition and execution of skills requiring motor coordination (Criterion A). Manifestations vary with age and stage of development. For example, younger children may display delays and clumsiness in achieving developmental motor milestones such as crawling, sitting, and walking, or in acquiring and using motor skills or tasks such as negotiating stairs, pedaling bicycles, buttoning shirts, and using zippers. Older children may display difficulties with motor aspects of assembling puzzles or building models.

Developmental coordination disorder is diagnosed when the impairment significantly and persistently interferes with the performance of or participation in daily activities in family, social, school, or community life (Criterion B). These include activities such as getting dressed, eating meals with appropriate utensils, engaging in physical games with peers, and participating in exercise activities at school. Typically, the child's ability to perform these actions is impaired, and there is a marked slowness in their execution. Consequences of this disorder can include reduced participation in team play and sports, low self-esteem and sense of self-worth, and emotional or behavioral problems. For adolescents and adults, impairment in fine motor skills and motor speed may affect performance in the workplace or school setting. Onset is in the early developmental period (Criterion C).

Developmental coordination disorder must be distinguished from other medical conditions that may produce coordination problems, such as cerebral palsy or muscular dystrophy, visual impairment, or intellectual disability (intellectual developmental disorder) (Criterion D).

---

### Diagnostic Criteria for Developmental Coordination Disorder                                    315.4 (F82)

A. The acquisition and execution of coordinated motor skills is substantially below that expected given the individual's chronological age and opportunity for skill learning and use. Difficulties are manifested as clumsiness (e.g., dropping or bumping into objects) as well as slowness and inaccuracy of performance of motor skills (e.g., catching an object, using scissors or cutlery, handwriting, riding a bike, or participating in sports).

B. The motor skills deficit in Criterion A significantly and persistently interferes with activities of daily living appropriate to chronological age (e.g., self-care and self-maintenance) and impacts academic/school productivity, prevocational and vocational activities, leisure, and play.

C. Onset of symptoms is in the early developmental period.

D. The motor skills deficits are not better explained by intellectual disability (intellectual developmental disorder) or visual impairment and are not attributable to a neurological condition affecting movement (e.g., cerebral palsy, muscular dystrophy, degenerative disorder).

# Stereotypic Movement Disorder

Stereotypic movement disorder is characterized by repetitive, seemingly driven, and apparently purposeless motor behavior (Criterion A) that interferes with social, academic, and other activities or results in self-injury (Criterion B). The disorder has an onset in the early developmental period (Criterion C). The behaviors are not attributable to the physiological effects of a substance or a neurological condition, and are not better explained by another neurodevelopmental or mental disorder (e.g., a compulsion as in obsessive-compulsive disorder, a tic as in a tic disorder, a stereotypy that is part of autism spectrum disorder, or hair pulling as in trichotillomania) (Criterion D). Typical movements include hand waving, rocking, playing with hands, fiddling with fingers, twirling objects, head banging, self-biting, and hitting various parts of one's own body. These behaviors may cause permanent and disabling tissue damage and may sometimes be life threatening.

Changes have been made in the criteria for DSM-5. Because the term *nonfunctional* (DSM-IV Criterion A) may be inaccurate, the wording "apparently purposeless" has been substituted. Because there is no evidence that the disorder must persist for 4 weeks or longer, that criterion (DSM-IV Criterion F) has been eliminated.

## Diagnostic Criteria for Stereotypic Movement Disorder　　　　**307.3** (F98.4)

A. Repetitive, seemingly driven, and apparently purposeless motor behavior (e.g., hand shaking or waving, body rocking, head banging, self-biting, hitting own body).
B. The repetitive motor behavior interferes with social, academic, or other activities and may result in self-injury.
C. Onset is in the early developmental period.
D. The repetitive motor behavior is not attributable to the physiological effects of a substance or neurological condition and is not better explained by another neurodevelopmental or mental disorder (e.g., trichotillomania [hair-pulling disorder], obsessive-compulsive disorder).

*Specify* if:
　　**With self-injurious behavior** (or behavior that would result in an injury if preventive measures were not used)
　　**Without self-injurious behavior**
*Specify* if:
　　**Associated with a known medical or genetic condition, neurodevelopmental disorder, or environmental factor** (e.g., Lesch-Nyhan syndrome, intellectual disability [intellectual developmental disorder], intrauterine alcohol exposure)

**Coding note:** Use additional code to identify the associated medical or genetic condition, or neurodevelopmental disorder.

*Specify* current severity:

**Mild:** Symptoms are easily suppressed by sensory stimulus or distraction.

**Moderate:** Symptoms require explicit protective measures and behavioral modification.

**Severe:** Continuous monitoring and protective measures are required to prevent serious injury.

# Tic Disorders

Tic disorders are characterized by the presence of clinically significant tics and differ mainly with respect to duration and type. The inclusion of five tic disorders—Tourette's disorder, persistent (chronic) motor or vocal tic disorder, provisional tic disorder, other specified tic disorder, and unspecified tic disorder—represents an expansion from the four listed in DSM-IV (Walkup et al. 2010). The latter two diagnoses were added based on research suggesting that tics may result from the effect of certain substances (e.g., cocaine) or medical conditions (e.g., Huntington's disease).

## Tourette's Disorder

Tourette's disorder is characterized by stereotypical but nonrhythmic motor movements and vocalizations. The vocal tics can be socially offensive, such as loud grunting or barking noises or shouted words, which may be obscenities. The individual is aware that he or she is producing the vocal tics and is able to exert a mild degree of control over them, but ultimately must submit to them. Because people with Tourette's disorder are aware that their tics are socially inappropriate, they find the tics embarrassing. Motor tics occurring in Tourette's disorder are also often odd or offensive behaviors, such as tongue protrusion, sniffing, hopping, squatting, blinking, or nodding. Because most of the general public is unaware of the nature of Tourette's disorder, the behavior is seen as inappropriate or bizarre.

---

Diagnostic Criteria for Tourette's Disorder                    **307.23** (F95.2)

---

**Note:** A tic is a sudden, rapid, recurrent, nonrhythmic motor movement or vocalization.
A. Both multiple motor and one or more vocal tics have been present at some time during the illness, although not necessarily concurrently.
B. The tics may wax and wane in frequency but have persisted for more than 1 year since first tic onset.
C. Onset is before age 18 years.
D. The disturbance is not attributable to the physiological effects of a substance (e.g., cocaine) or another medical condition (e.g., Huntington's disease, postviral encephalitis).

**Criterion A.** The definition of a tic has been made consistent for all tic disorders. The term *stereotyped* has been removed to make it less likely that individuals with stereotypic movement disorder will be diagnosed with a tic disorder.

**Criterion B.** The maximum tic-free interval (DSM-IV Criterion B) was eliminated because there are no data to suggest that tic-free periods of more than 3 months do *not* constitute a chronic course. Also, tic-free intervals are more difficult to assess because they require the patient to recall offset of symptoms, and this may lead to unreliability in diagnosis. DSM-5 maintains that tics must have persisted for more than 1 year, as in DSM-IV, but it clarifies that the 12-month duration of symptoms is since first tic onset. The phrase "usually in bouts" was eliminated because this feature of tics is not critical to diagnosis.

**Criteria C and D.** The tics must be present before age 18 years. This requirement helps distinguish Tourette's disorder from other causes of tics that occur later in life, such as Huntington's disease or postviral encephalitis. Stimulant medication use as an example of a substance-induced movement disorder is not consistent with the evidence base and has been eliminated. Cocaine has been substituted as an example.

## Persistent (Chronic) Motor or Vocal Tic Disorder

The essential feature of persistent (chronic) motor or vocal tic disorder is the presence of either motor tics or vocal tics, but not both. This disorder differs from Tourette's disorder, for which diagnosis requires *both* multiple motor tics and one or more vocal tics. The other features are the same as for Tourette's disorder, such as onset before age 18 years. Other disorders, such as Huntington's disease, need to be ruled out as causes. The diagnosis cannot be made if the criteria for Tourette's disorder have ever been met. The other characteristics are generally the same as for Tourette's disorder except that the severity of the symptoms and the functional impairment are usually much less. Persistent (chronic) motor or vocal tic disorder and Tourette's disorder may be genetically related. Clinicians can specify whether the disorder is "with motor tics only" or "with vocal tics only."

---

Diagnostic Criteria for Persistent (Chronic)
Motor or Vocal Tic Disorder                                    **307.22** (F95.1)

---

**Note:** A tic is a sudden, rapid, recurrent, nonrhythmic motor movement or vocalization.
A. Single or multiple motor or vocal tics have been present during the illness, but not both motor and vocal.
B. The tics may wax and wane in frequency but have persisted for more than 1 year since first tic onset.
C. Onset is before age 18 years.
D. The disturbance is not attributable to the physiological effects of a substance (e.g., cocaine) or another medical condition (e.g., Huntington's disease, postviral encephalitis).

E. Criteria have never been met for Tourette's disorder.

*Specify* if:

**With motor tics only**

**With vocal tics only**

---

**Criteria A and B.**   The definition of a tic has been made consistent with that used in the other tic disorders. The changes to Criterion B for persistent (chronic) motor or vocal tic disorder are identical to those for Tourette's disorder.

**Criteria C and D.**   Onset must occur before age 18. This requirement helps separate the disorder from other causes of tics that occur later in life, such as Huntington's disease or postviral encephalitis. Stimulant medication use as an example of a substance-induced movement disorder has been removed. Cocaine has been substituted as an example.

## Provisional Tic Disorder

The provisional tic disorder diagnosis represents a modification of transient tic disorder in DSM-IV. The DSM-IV criteria were difficult to use because individuals with current tic symptoms of less than 1 year's duration would be diagnosed as having transient tics when the tics were actually present. Given the need for a diagnostic category for persons with tics of less than 1 year's duration, the transient tic disorder category has been renamed *provisional tic disorder.*

---

### Diagnostic Criteria for Provisional Tic Disorder       **307.21** (F95.0)

---

**Note:** A tic is a sudden, rapid, recurrent, nonrhythmic motor movement or vocalization.

A. Single or multiple motor and/or vocal tics.

B. The tics have been present for less than 1 year since first tic onset.

C. Onset is before age 18 years.

D. The disturbance is not attributable to the physiological effects of a substance (e.g., cocaine) or another medical condition (e.g., Huntington's disease, postviral encephalitis).

E. Criteria have never been met for Tourette's disorder or persistent (chronic) motor or vocal tic disorder.

---

**Criteria A, B, C, and D.**   The definition of a tic has been made consistent with that used in the other tic disorders. No evidence suggests that the 4-week threshold described in DSM-IV was valid or useful, so it has been omitted. Onset must occur before age 18; this helps separate the disorder from other causes of tics that occur later in life, such as Huntington's disease or postviral encephalitis. Stimulant medication use as an example of a substance-induced movement disorder has been removed. Cocaine has been substituted as an example.

# Other Specified Tic Disorder and Unspecified Tic Disorder

Other specified tic disorder is a diagnosis used when an impairing tic disorder is present, but the full criteria for a specific tic disorder or any of the disorders in the neurodevelopmental disorders diagnostic class are not met. Unspecified tic disorder is used when the above conditions are present, but the clinician chooses not to specify the reason that the criteria are not met for a specific disorder, and includes presentations in which there is insufficient information to make a more specific diagnosis. These two diagnoses replace DSM-IV's tic disorder not otherwise specified.

## Other Specified Tic Disorder                      **307.20** (F95.8)

This category applies to presentations in which symptoms characteristic of a tic disorder that cause clinically significant distress or impairment in social, occupational, or other important areas of functioning predominate but do not meet the full criteria for a tic disorder or any of the disorders in the neurodevelopmental disorders diagnostic class. The other specified tic disorder category is used in situations in which the clinician chooses to communicate the specific reason that the presentation does not meet the criteria for a tic disorder or any specific neurodevelopmental disorder. This is done by recording "other specified tic disorder" followed by the specific reason (e.g., "with onset after age 18 years").

## Unspecified Tic Disorder                         **307.20** (F95.9)

This category applies to presentations in which symptoms characteristic of a tic disorder that cause clinically significant distress or impairment in social, occupational, or other important areas of functioning predominate but do not meet the full criteria for a tic disorder or for any of the disorders in the neurodevelopmental disorders diagnostic class. The unspecified tic disorder category is used in situations in which the clinician chooses *not* to specify the reason that the criteria are not met for a tic disorder or for a specific neurodevelopmental disorder, and includes presentations in which there is insufficient information to make a more specific diagnosis.

# Other Neurodevelopmental Disorders

## Other Specified Neurodevelopmental Disorder and Unspecified Neurodevelopmental Disorder

These categories apply to presentations in which symptoms characteristic of a neurodevelopmental disorder are present and impairing but do not meet the full criteria for any of the disorders in the neurodevelopmental disorders diagnostic class. The other specified neurodevelopmental disorder category is used when the clinician chooses to communicate the reason that the presentation does not meet the criteria. The unspecified neurodevelopmental disorder category is used when the clinician chooses not to specify the reason, or there is insufficient information to make a more specific diagnosis.

### Other Specified Neurodevelopmental Disorder          315.8 (F88)

This category applies to presentations in which symptoms characteristic of a neurodevelopmental disorder that cause impairment in social, occupational, or other important areas of functioning predominate but do not meet the full criteria for any of the disorders in the neurodevelopmental disorders diagnostic class. The other specified neurodevelopmental disorder category is used in situations in which the clinician chooses to communicate the specific reason that the presentation does not meet the criteria for any specific neurodevelopmental disorder. This is done by recording "other specified neurodevelopmental disorder" followed by the specific reason (e.g., "neurodevelopmental disorder associated with prenatal alcohol exposure").

An example of a presentation that can be specified using the "other specified" designation is the following:

**Neurodevelopmental disorder associated with prenatal alcohol exposure:** Neurodevelopmental disorder associated with prenatal alcohol exposure is characterized by a range of developmental disabilities following exposure to alcohol in utero.

### Unspecified Neurodevelopmental Disorder          315.9 (F89)

This category applies to presentations in which symptoms characteristic of a neurodevelopmental disorder that cause impairment in social, occupational, or other important areas of functioning predominate but do not meet the full criteria for any of the disorders in the neurodevelopmental disorders diagnostic class. The unspecified neurodevelopmental disorder category is used in situations in which the clinician chooses *not* to specify the reason that the criteria are not met for a specific neurodevelopmental disorder, and includes presentations in which there is insufficient information to make a more specific diagnosis (e.g., in emergency room settings).

# KEY POINTS

- The chapter on neurodevelopmental disorders is a reformulation of the DSM-IV chapter "Disorders Usually First Diagnosed in Infancy, Childhood, or Adolescence."

- Mental retardation has been renamed *intellectual disability (intellectual developmental disorder)*. Severity is determined on the basis of adaptive functioning rather than an IQ score, though diagnostic criteria emphasize the need to assess cognitive capacity.

- The communication disorders are newly named and include language disorder (which combines expressive and mixed receptive-expressive language disorders), speech sound disorder (previously phonological disorder), and childhood-onset fluency disorder (previously stuttering). Social (pragmatic) communication disorder is new and describes persistent difficulties in the social uses of verbal and nonverbal communication.

- Autism spectrum disorder is a new diagnosis that now subsumes DSM-IV autistic disorder, Rett's disorder, childhood disintegrative disorder, Asperger's disorder, and pervasive developmental disorder not otherwise specified. Work group members believed that there was little validity to the specific diagnoses and that clinicians had difficulty distinguishing them.

- With attention-deficit/hyperactivity disorder, examples have been added to the criterion items to enhance use of these items across the life span. Age at onset has been changed from before age 7 years to before age 12 years. A comorbid diagnosis with autism spectrum disorder is now allowed. Last, the symptom threshold has been changed for adults, with a cutoff of five symptoms instead of the six required for younger persons, both for inattention and for hyperactivity and impulsivity.

- DSM-IV learning disorder has been changed to *specific learning disorder*. The previous types of learning disorders (reading disorder, mathematics disorder, and disorder of written expression) have been combined, and specifiers are now used to describe the individual's impairment.

- With tic disorders, the maximum tic-free interval (DSM-IV Criterion B) was eliminated because there are no scientific data to suggest that tic-free periods of more than 3 months do *not* constitute a chronic course.

# References

American Psychiatric Association: Diagnostic and Statistical Manual of Mental Disorders, 2nd Edition. Washington, DC, American Psychiatric Association, 1968

Applegate B, Lahey BB, Hart EL, et al: Validity of the age-of-onset criterion for ADHD: a report from the DSM-IV field trials. J Am Acad Child Adolesc Psychiatry 36:1211–1221, 1997

Bishop DVM: Pragmatic language impairment: a correlate of SLI, a distinct subgroup, or part of the autistic continuum? in Speech and Language Impairments in Children: Causes, Characteristics, Intervention, and Outcome. Edited by Bishop DVM, Leonard LB. East Sussex, UK, Psychology Press, 2000, pp 99–113

Bishop DV, Norbury CF: Exploring the borderlands of autistic disorder and specific language impairment: a study using standardised diagnostic instruments. J Child Psychol Psychiatry 43:917–929, 2002

Kieling C, Kieling RR, Rohde LA, et al: The age at onset of attention deficit hyperactivity disorder. Am J Psychiatry 167:14–16, 2010

Matte B, Rohde LA, Grevet EH: ADHD in adults: a concept in evolution. Atten Defic Hyperact Disord 4:53–62, 2012

Walkup JT, Ferrao Y, Leckman JF, et al: Tic disorders: some key issues for DSM-V. Depress Anxiety 27:600–610, 2010

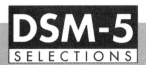

# Neurodevelopmental Disorders

## DSM-5® Clinical Cases

## Introduction

*Robert Haskell, M.D.*

In its approach to mental illness across the lifetime of a patient, DSM-5 naturally begins with the neurodevelopmental disorders. As a group, these disorders are usually first diagnosed in infancy, childhood, or adolescence. Individually, these disorders have undergone a mix of pruning, reorganization, and clarification, including one of DSM-5's most controversial changes—to the definition of and diagnostic criteria for autism.

In DSM-5, autism spectrum disorder describes patients previously divided among autistic disorder, Asperger's disorder, childhood disintegrative disorder, Rett's disorder, and pervasive developmental disorder not otherwise specified. These are no longer considered to be separate clinical entities. The new criteria include 1) persistent and pervasive deficits in social communication and social interaction and 2) restricted, repetitive patterns of behavior, interests, and activities. As now defined, autism spectrum disorder (ASD) can be subcategorized by the presence or absence of intellectual impairment and/or an associated medical condition. In addition, the identification of three severity levels helps clarify the need for additional social or occupational services. For example, a patient requiring "very substantial support" might display extreme behavioral inflexibility or might possess 20 words of intelligible speech.

Attention-deficit/hyperactivity disorder (ADHD) continues to be subdivided into two symptom dimensions (inattention and hyperactivity/impulsivity), with a core requirement being the presence of at least six symptoms from either or both of the two dimensions. For example, inattention might be noted by the presence of such behaviors as making careless mistakes, failing to follow through with homework, and losing books. Criteria for hyperactivity/impulsivity include fidgetiness, impatience, and garrulousness. The diagnosis of ADHD is generally incomplete without inclusion of dimensional specifiers (predominantly inattentive, predominantly hyperactive/impulsive, or combined). Several of these symptoms must have been present prior to age 12, a change from DSM-IV's requirement that symptoms causing impairment be present prior to age 7. Another change is a reduction in the number of symptomatic criteria for adults from six to five within a particular dimension. These latter two changes reflect evidence that "loosening" criteria allows for identification of people who have symptoms, distress, and dysfunction that are very similar to those of people already diagnosed with ADHD and who can potentially benefit from clinical attention. As is true throughout DSM-5, it is up to the clinician to diagnose only those people who meet symptomatic criteria and whose distress and dysfunction reach a relevant clinical threshold.

Falling in line with both federal legislative language and the words used by sensitive practitioners, DSM-5 has replaced the term *mental retardation* with *intellectual disability.* The three core criteria are unchanged: deficits in intellectual function and in adaptation (in areas such as communication, work, or leisure), as well as an early age at onset. The diagnosis no longer depends, however, on formal intelligence testing. Instead, DSM-5 invites the clinician to make an aggregate assessment of severity, from mild to profound, according to three important life domains: conceptual, social, and practical. For example, a person with severe intellectual disability might have little understanding of concepts like time or money, might use language to communicate but not to explain, and would likely require support for all activities of daily living.

Disorders of communication first observed in childhood include language disorder (formerly divided into expressive and receptive language disorders); speech-sound disorder, in which the patient displays an impaired ability to produce the phonological building blocks of words but has no congenital or acquired medical condition that explains the impairment; childhood-onset fluency disorder (stuttering); and a new diagnosis, social (pragmatic) communication disorder, in which the patient displays persistent difficulties in the social use of verbal and nonverbal communication—very likely a diagnostic home for some of the individuals who have traits of ASD but do not meet full criteria.

Specific learning disorder is a new umbrella diagnosis within DSM-5. Specifiers for reading, written expression, and mathematics are designed to help teachers and parents shine a more focused light on a child's academic needs.

The chapter on neurodevelopmental disorders culminates with the motor disorders, including developmental coordination disorder, stereotypic movement disorder, and the tic disorders. A tic is a nonrhythmic movement of short duration and sudden onset. Such movements can be divided into motor tics, such as shoulder shrugs and eyeblinks, and vocal tics, including sniffs, snorts, and the spontaneous production of a word or phrase. Tourette's disorder is the most complex of the tic disorders, describing patients who exhibit both multiple motor and at least one vocal tic for more than 1 year that cannot be explained by a medical condition or by the physiological effects of a substance such as cocaine.

Inevitably, the neurodevelopmental disorders share symptoms with a broad range of psychiatric illnesses, and clinicians must sort through the differential diagnosis with an understanding that that differential is much broader for children age 12 and under. Sometimes the neurodevelopmental disorders contribute to the emergence of other disorders; for example, a learning disorder may cause anxiety, and untreated ADHD may make a patient vulnerable to substance abuse. The cases that follow attempt to pull apart some of these diagnostic entanglements and explore the comorbidities that make the treatment of neurodevelopmental disorders among the most challenging tasks in psychiatry.

## Suggested Readings

Brown TE (ed): ADHD Comorbidities. Washington, DC, American Psychiatric Publishing, 2009

Hansen RL, Rogers SJ (eds): Autism and Other Neurodevelopmental Disorders. Washington, DC, American Psychiatric Publishing, 2013

Tanguay PE: Autism in DSM-5. Am J Psychiatry 168(11):1142–1144, 2011

# Case 1: A Second Opinion on Autism

*Catherine Lord, Ph.D.*

Ashley, age 17, was referred for a diagnostic reevaluation after having carried diagnoses of autism and mental retardation for almost all of her life. She was recently found to have Kleefstra syndrome, and the family would like to reconfirm the earlier diagnoses and assess the genetic risk to the future children of her older sisters.

At the time of the reevaluation, Ashley was attending a special school with a focus on functional skills. She was able to dress herself, but she was not able to shower independently or be left alone in the house. She was able to decode (e.g., read words) and spell at a second-grade level but understood little of what she read. Changes to her schedule and heightened functional expectations tended to make her irritable. When upset, Ashley would often hurt herself (e.g., biting her wrist) and others (e.g., pinching and hair pulling).

In formal testing done at the time of the reevaluation, Ashley had a nonverbal IQ of 39 and a verbal IQ of 23, with a full scale IQ of 31. Her adaptive scores were somewhat higher, with an overall score of 42 (with 100 as average).

By history, Ashley first received services at age 9 months after her parents noticed significant motor delays. She walked at 20 months and was toilet trained at 5 years. She spoke her first word at age 6. She received a diagnosis of developmental delay at age 3 and of autism, obesity, and static encephalopathy at age 4. An early evaluation noted possible facial dysmorphology; genetic tests at that time were noncontributory.

Her parents indicated that Ashley knew hundreds of single words and many simple phrases. She had long been very interested in license plates and would draw them for hours. Her strongest skill was memory, and she could draw precise representations of license plates from different states. Ashley had always been very attached to her parents and sisters, and although affectionate toward babies, she showed minimal interest in other teenagers.

Ashley's family history was pertinent for a father with dyslexia, a paternal uncle with epilepsy, and a maternal male cousin with possible "Asperger's syndrome." Her siblings, both sisters, were in college and doing well.

On examination, Ashley was an overweight young woman who made inconsistent eye contact but often peered out the corner of her eye. She had a beautiful smile and would sometimes laugh to herself, but most of the time her facial expressions were subdued. She did not initiate joint attention by trying to catch another person's eyes. She frequently ignored what others would say to her. To request a preferred object (e.g., a shiny magazine), Ashley would rock from foot to foot and point. When offered an object (e.g., a stuffed animal), she brought it to her nose and lips for inspection. Ashley spoke in a high-pitched voice with unusual intonation. During the interview, she used multiple words and a few short phrases that were somewhat rote but communicative, such as "I want to clean up," and "Do you have a van?"

In the months prior to the evaluation, Ashley's parents noticed that she had become increasingly apathetic. A medical evaluation concluded that urinary tract infections were the most likely cause for her symptoms, but antibiotics seemed only to make her more listless. Further medical evaluation led to more extensive genetic testing, and Ashley was diagnosed with Kleefstra syndrome, a rare genetic defect associated with multiple medical problems including intellectual disability. The parents said they were also checked and found to "be negative."

The parents specifically wanted to know whether the genetic testing results affected Ashley's long-standing diagnoses and access to future services. Furthermore, they wanted to know whether their other two daughters should get tested for their risk of carrying genes for autism, mental retardation, and/or Kleefstra syndrome.

## Diagnoses

- Intellectual disability, severe
- Autism spectrum disorder (ASD), with accompanying intellectual and language impairments, associated with Kleefstra syndrome

## Discussion

In regard to diagnosis, Ashley's cognitive testing and limited everyday adaptive skills indicate that she has DSM-5 intellectual disability. In addition, Ashley has prominent symptoms from both of the core symptomatic criteria of ASD: 1) deficits in social communication and 2) restricted, repetitive patterns of behavior, interests, or activities. Ashley also fulfills the DSM-5 ASD requirement of having had symptoms in the early developmental period and a history of significant impairment. A fifth requirement for ASD is that the disturbances are not better explained by intellectual disability, which is a more complicated question in Ashley's case.

For many years, clinicians and researchers have debated the boundary between autism and intellectual disabilities. As IQ decreases, the proportion of children and adults who meet criteria for autism increases. Most individuals with IQs below 30 have ASD as well as intellectual disability.

For Ashley to meet DSM-5 criteria for both ASD and intellectual disability, the specific deficits and behaviors associated with ASD must be greater than what would ordinarily be seen in people with her overall intellectual development. In other words, if her deficits were due solely to limited intellectual abilities, she would be expected to have the social and play skills of a typical 3- to 4-year-old child. Ashley's social interaction is not at all like that of a typical preschooler, however, and never has been. She has limited facial expressions, poor eye contact, and minimal interest in peers. Compared to her "mental age," Ashley demonstrates significant restriction in both her range of interests and her understanding of basic human emotions. Furthermore, she manifests behaviors that are not seen commonly at any age.

The heterogeneity of autism has led to significant conflict. Some argue, for example, that children with very severe intellectual disabilities should be excluded from ASD. Others argue that more intellectually able children with ASD should be placed into their own category, Asperger syndrome. Research does not support either of these distinctions. For example, studies indicate that children with autistic symptoms and severe intellectual disability often have siblings with autism and stronger intellectual abilities. Much remains to be known about ASD, but IQ does not appear to be the key distinguishing factor.

From a pragmatic perspective, the critical factor is whether an ASD diagnosis offers information that helps guide treatment and the availability of services. For Ashley, the ASD diagnosis encourages a focus on her poor social skills. It calls attention to differences in her motivation and in her need for structure. The ASD diagnosis also underlines the importance of looking carefully for her cognitive strengths (e.g., rote memory and visual representation) and weaknesses (e.g., comprehension, social interaction, and an ability to adapt to change). All of these may play a large role in her efforts to live as independently as possible.

Ashley's parents are also concerned about the impact of the recent genetic testing results on Ashley's treatment and on her sisters' family planning. Hundreds of individual genes may play a role in the complex neurological issues involved in autism, but most cases of ASD lack a clear cause. Ashley's genetic condition, Kleefstra syndrome, is reliably associated with both intellectual disability and ASD symptoms. When a genetic or medical condition or environmental factor appears to be implicated, it is listed as a specifier, but the ASD diagnosis is not otherwise affected.

Knowledge of the genetic cause for Ashley's intellectual disability and ASD is important for several reasons. It reminds her physicians to look for medical comorbidities that are common in Kleefstra syndrome, such as problems with the heart and kidneys (possibly leading, for example, to her recurrent urinary tract infections). Knowledge of the genetic cause also expands informational resources by connecting Ashley's family to other families that are affected by this rare syndrome.

A particularly important aspect of this new genetic diagnosis is its effect on Ashley's sisters. In almost all reported cases, Kleefstra syndrome has occurred de novo, meaning that there is an extremely low likelihood that anyone else in her family has any abnormality in the affected gene region. On rare occasions, an unaffected parent has a chromosomal translocation or mosaicism that leads to the syndrome, but the fact that Ashley's parents were found to "be negative" implies they are not genetic carriers. Although this is not necessarily true for situations involving other autism-related genetic disorders, this particular genetic diagnosis in Ashley likely indicates her sisters are not at increased risk for having children with autism. Such information can be very reassuring and useful to Ashley's sisters. The fact remains that although genetics undoubtedly plays a large role in autism and intellectual disability, most cases cannot be reliably predicted, and diagnosis is made through ongoing, longitudinal observation during childhood.

## Suggested Readings

Kleefstra T, Nillesen WM, Yntema HG: Kleefstra syndrome. GeneReviews October 5, 2010

Lord C, Pickles A: Language level and nonverbal social-communicative behaviors in autistic and language-delayed children. J Am Acad Child Adolesc Psychiatry 35(11):1542–1550, 1996

Lord C, Spence SJ: Autism spectrum disorders: phenotype and diagnosis, in Understanding Autism: From Basic Neuroscience to Treatment. Edited by Moldin SO, Rubenstein JLR. Boca Raton, FL, Taylor & Francis, 2006, pp 1–24

Shattuck PT, Durkin M, Maenner M, et al: Timing of identification among children with an autism spectrum disorder: findings from a population-based surveillance study. J Am Acad Child Adolesc Psychiatry 48(5):474–483, 2009

Wing L, Gould J: Severe impairments of social interaction and associated abnormalities in children: epidemiology and classification. J Autism Dev Disord 9(1):11–29, 1979

# Case 2: Temper Tantrums

*Arshya Vahabzadeh, M.D.*
*Eugene Beresin, M.D.*
*Christopher McDougle, M.D.*

Brandon was a 12-year-old boy brought in by his mother for psychiatric evaluation for temper tantrums that seemed to be contributing to declining school performance. The mother became emotional as she reported that things had always been difficult but had become worse after Brandon entered middle school.

Brandon's sixth-grade teachers reported that he was academically capable but that he had little ability to make friends. He seemed to mistrust the intentions of classmates who tried to be nice to him, and then trusted others who laughingly feigned interest in the toy cars and trucks that he brought to school. The teachers noted that he often cried and rarely spoke in class. In recent months, multiple teachers had heard him screaming at other boys, generally in the hallway but sometimes in the middle of class. The teachers had not identified a cause but generally had not disciplined Brandon because they assumed he was responding to provocation.

When interviewed alone, Brandon responded with nonspontaneous mumbles when asked questions about school, classmates, and his family. When the examiner asked if he was interested in toy cars, however, Brandon lit up. He pulled several cars, trucks, and airplanes from his backpack and, while not making good eye contact, did talk at length about vehicles, using their apparently accurate names (e.g., front-end loader, B-52, Jaguar). When asked again about school, Brandon pulled out his cell phone and showed a string of text messages: "dumbo!!!!, mr stutter, LoSeR, freak!, EVERYBODY HATES YOU." While the examiner read the long string of texts that Brandon had saved but apparently not previously revealed, Brandon added that other boys would whisper "bad words" to him in class and then scream in his ears in the hall. "And I hate loud noises." He said he had considered running away, but then had decided that maybe he should just run away to his own bedroom.

Developmentally, Brandon spoke his first word at age 11 months and began to use short sentences by age 3. He had always been very focused on trucks, cars, and trains. According to his mother, he had always been "very shy" and had never had a best friend. He struggled with jokes and typical childhood banter because "he takes things so literally." Brandon's mother had long seen this behavior as "a little odd" but added that it was not much different from that of Brandon's father, a successful attorney, who had similarly focused interests. Both of them were "sticklers for routine" who "lacked a sense of humor."

On examination, Brandon was shy and generally nonspontaneous. He made below-average eye contact. His speech was coherent and goal directed. At times, Brandon stumbled over his words, paused excessively, and sometimes rapidly repeated words or parts of words. Brandon said he felt okay but added he was scared of school. He appeared sad, brightening only when discussing his toy cars. He denied suicidality and homicidality. He denied psychotic symptoms. He was cognitively intact.

## Diagnosis

- Autism spectrum disorder without accompanying intellectual impairment, with accompanying language impairment: childhood-onset fluency disorder (stuttering)

## Discussion

Brandon presents with symptoms consistent with autism spectrum disorder (ASD), a new diagnosis in DSM-5. ASD incorporates several previously separate disorders, namely autistic disorder (autism), Asperger's disorder, and pervasive developmental disorder not otherwise specified. ASD is characterized by two main symptom domains: social communication deficits and a fixated set of interests and repetitive behaviors.

It is evident that Brandon has considerable difficulty in his peer social interactions. He is unable to form friendships, does not engage in interactive play, and struggles with reading social cues. People with ASD typically find it challenging to correctly interpret the relevance of facial expressions, body language, and other nonverbal behaviors. He is humorless and "takes things so literally." These symptoms meet the ASD criteria for social communication deficits.

In regard to the second ASD symptom domain, Brandon has fixated interests and repetitive behaviors that cause significant distress. He seems interested in cars and trains, has little interest in anything else, and has no apparent insight that other children might not share his enthusiasms. He requires "sameness," with distress arising if his routine is altered. Brandon meets both of the primary symptomatic criteria, therefore, for DSM-5 ASD.

Brandon also stumbles over his words, pauses excessively, and repeats words or parts of words. These symptoms are consistent with stuttering, which is classified as one of the DSM-5 communication disorders, namely childhood-onset fluency disorder. Typically persistent and characterized by frequent repetitions or prolongations of sounds, broken words, pauses in speech, and circumlocutions, childhood-onset fluency disorder may result in significant social, academic, and occupational dysfunction.

Other DSM-5 communication disorders include difficulties in speech production (speech sound disorder), difficulty in use of spoken and written language (language disorder), and difficulty in the social uses of verbal and nonverbal communication (social [pragmatic] communication disorder). Although these difficulties are not noted in the case report, Brandon should be evaluated for each of these, because language impairments are so commonly part of ASD that they are listed as specifiers of ASD rather than as separate, comorbid diagnoses.

Prior to DSM-5, Brandon would have met criteria for Asperger's disorder, which identified a cluster of individuals with core autism features (social deficits and fixated interests) and normal intelligence. Perhaps because he shared autism spectrum symptoms with his own father, however, Brandon was viewed as "a little odd" but without problems that merited specific clinical attention. The lack of a diagnosis contributed to Brandon's having become the defenseless target of malicious bullying, a not uncommon finding in people with ASD. Without appropriate interventions for both his core autism symptoms and his stuttering, Brandon is at serious risk for ongoing psychological trauma and academic derailment.

## Suggested Readings

Sterzing PR, Shattuck PT, Narendorf SC, et al: Bullying involvement and autism spectrum disorders: prevalence and correlates of bullying involvement among adolescents with an autism spectrum disorder. Arch Pediatr Adolesc Med 166(11):1058–1064, 2012
Toth K, King BH: Asperger's syndrome: diagnosis and treatment. Am J Psychiatry 165(8):958–963, 2008

# Case 3: Academic Difficulties

*Rosemary Tannock, Ph.D.*

Carlos, a 19-year-old Hispanic college student, presented to a primary care clinic for help with academic difficulties. Since starting college 6 months earlier, he had done poorly on tests and been unable to manage his study schedule. His worries that he was going to flunk out of college were leading to insomnia, poor concentration, and a general sense of hopelessness. After a particularly tough week, he returned home unexpectedly, telling his family that he thought he should quit. His mother quickly brought him to the clinic that had previously helped both Carlos and his older brother. The mother specifically wondered whether Carlos's "ADHD" might be causing his problems, or whether he had outgrown it.

Carlos had been seen at the same clinic when he was age 9, at which time he had been diagnosed with attention-deficit/hyperactivity disorder (ADHD), predominantly combined type. Notes from that clinical evaluation indicated that Carlos had been in trouble at school for not following instructions, not completing homework, getting out of his seat, losing things, not waiting his turn, and not listening. He had trouble concentrating except in regard to video games, which he "could play for hours." Carlos had apparently been slow to talk, but his birth and developmental histories were otherwise normal. The family had immigrated to the United States from Mexico when Carlos was age 5. He repeated first grade because of behavioral immaturity and difficulty learning to read. The ease with which Carlos learned English, his second language, was not noted.

During the evaluation when Carlos was age 9, a psychoeducational assessment by a clinical psychologist confirmed reading problems (particularly problems in reading fluency and comprehension). Carlos did not, however, meet the school board criteria for learning disability, which required evidence of a 20-point discrepancy between IQ and achievement scores. Thus, he was not eligible for special education services. Carlos's primary care physician had recommended pharmacotherapy, but the mother did not want to pursue medication. Instead, she reported taking on an extra job to pay for tutors to help her son "with concentration and reading."

Since starting college, Carlos reported that he had frequently been unable to remain focused while reading and listening to lectures. He was easily sidetracked and therefore had difficulty handing in his written assignments on time. He complained of feeling restless, agitated, and worried. He described difficulty falling asleep, poor energy, and an inability to "have fun" like his peers. He reported that the depressive symptoms went "up and down" over the course of the week but did not seem to influence his problems with concentration. He denied substance use.

Carlos said that he'd had some great teachers in high school who had understood him, helped him get the meaning of what he read, and allowed him to audiotape lectures and use other formats (e.g., videos, wikis, visual presentations) for final assignments. Without this support at college, he said he felt "lonely, stupid, a failure—unable to cope."

Although advised by his high school teacher to do so, he had not registered with the university's student disability services office. He preferred not to be seen as different from his peers and thought he should be able to get through college by himself.

Carlos's family history was positive for ADHD in his older brother. His father, who died when Carlos was age 7, was reported to have had "dyslexia" and had dropped out of a local community college after one semester.

On examination, Carlos wore clean jeans, a T-shirt, and a hoodie that he kept pulling down over his face. He sat quietly and hunched over. He sighed a lot and rarely made eye contact with the clinician. He often tapped his fingers and shuffled in his seat but was polite and responded appropriately to questions. His command of English appeared strong, but he spoke with a slight Hispanic accent. He often mumbled and mispronounced some multisyllabic words (e.g., he said "literalchure" instead of "literature" and "intimate" when he clearly meant "intimidate"). He denied any suicidal thoughts. He appeared to have reasonable insight into his problems.

Carlos was referred to a psychologist for further testing. The psychoeducational reassessment confirmed that Carlos's reading and writing abilities were substantially and quantifiably below those expected for his age. That report also concluded that these learning difficulties were not attributable to intellectual disability, uncorrected visual or auditory acuity, psychosocial adversity, or lack of proficiency in the language of academic instruction. The report concluded that Carlos had specific difficulties with reading fluency and comprehension as well as spelling and written expression.

## Diagnoses

- Attention-deficit/hyperactivity disorder, with predominantly inattentive presentation, of mild to moderate severity
- Specific learning disorder, affecting the domains of reading (both fluency and comprehension) and written expression (spelling and organization of written expression), all currently of moderate severity

## Discussion

Carlos presents with a history of ADHD. When he was first evaluated at age 9, DSM-IV criteria for ADHD required six of the nine symptoms listed in either of the two categories: inattention or hyperactivity-impulsivity (as well as an onset before age 12). He had been diagnosed as having the combined type of ADHD, indicating the specialty clinic had found at least six symptoms in each of these spheres.

Carlos now presents at age 19, and the case report indicates that he has five different inattentive symptoms and two symptoms related to hyperactivity-impulsivity. This seems to indicate a symptomatic improvement. Partial remission of ADHD is common with age, especially in regard to hyperactivity symptoms. Under DSM-IV, Carlos's ADHD would be said to have remitted. DSM-5, however, has a lower threshold of five symptoms in either category, rather than six. Carlos, therefore, does meet this diagnostic criterion for ADHD.

It is important to look for alternative explanations to ADHD, however, and one possibility is that his current symptoms might be better explained by mood disorder. During the past 6 months, Carlos has manifested anxious and depressive symptoms, but his inattention and poor concentration are apparently not restricted to or exacerbated by these episodes. His ADHD symptoms are chronic, and he had an onset during childhood without any concurrent mood or anxiety disorders. Moreover, his presenting symptoms of depression seem to have persisted only about 1 week, whereas his school difficulties are chronic.

Academic problems are common in ADHD even in the absence of a specific learning disorder (SLD), although SLDs are also commonly comorbid with ADHD. Even before his repeat psychological testing, Carlos appeared to have multiple historical issues that increase the likelihood of an SLD. His speech was delayed in his first language, Spanish; his reading was slow in both Spanish and English; and he received (and thrived with) educational accommodations in high school. All of these suggest an SLD, as does his positive family history for learning disability.

Carlos's previous psychoeducational assessment failed to confirm a learning disorder because he did not meet the required discrepancy between IQ and achievement for diagnosis with an SLD. Based on an additional decade of evidence, DSM-5 has eliminated this discrepancy criterion for SLD. This change has made it reasonable to refer older adolescent patients for reevaluation.

The repeat psychological testing indicates a moderately severe SLD. Because Carlos's learning difficulties began when he was school age and continue to cause academic impairment, he meets the DSM-5 diagnostic criteria for SLD. By providing documentation of both ADHD and SLD, Carlos will be able to access academic accommodations that should allow him to more robustly pursue his college studies.

## Suggested Readings

Frazier TW, Youngstrom EA, Glutting JJ, Watkins MW: ADHD and achievement: meta-analysis of the child, adolescent, and adult literatures and a concomitant study with college students. J Learn Disabil 40(1):49–65, 2007

Sexton CC, Gelhorn H, Bell JA, Classi PM: The co-occurrence of reading disorder and ADHD: epidemiology, treatment, psychosocial impact, and economic burden. J Learn Disabil 45(6):538–564, 2012

Svetaz MV, Ireland M, Blum R: Adolescents with learning disabilities: risk and protective factors associated with emotional well-being: findings from the National Longitudinal Study of Adolescent Health. J Adolesc Health 27(5):340–348, 2000

Turgay A, Goodman DW, Asherson P, et al: Lifespan persistence of ADHD: the life transition model and its applications. J Clin Psychiatry 73(2):192–201, 2012

# Case 4: School Problems

*Arden Dingle, M.D.*

Daphne, a 13-year-old in the ninth grade, was brought for a psychiatric evaluation because of academic and behavioral struggles. She had particular difficulty starting and completing schoolwork and following instructions, and she had received failing grades in math. When prompted to complete tasks, Daphne became argumentative and irritable. She had become increasingly resistant to attending school, asking to stay home with her mother.

Testing indicated that Daphne had above-average intelligence, age-appropriate achievement in all subjects except math, and some difficulties in spatial-visual skills. Several years earlier, her pediatrician had diagnosed attention-deficit/hyperactivity disorder (ADHD) and prescribed a stimulant. She took the medication for a week, but her parents stopped giving it to her because she seemed agitated.

At home, Daphne's parents' close supervision of her homework often led to arguments with crying and screaming. She had two long-standing friends but had made no new friends for several years. Generally, she preferred to play with girls younger than she. When her friends chose the activity or did not follow her rules, she tended to withdraw. She was generally quiet in groups and in school but bolder with family members.

Beginning in early childhood, Daphne had had difficulty falling asleep, requiring a nightlight and parental reassurance. Recognizing that Daphne was easily upset by change, her parents rarely forced her into new activities. She did well during the summer, which she spent at a lake house with her grandparents. Her parents reported no particular traumas, stressors, or medical or developmental problems. Daphne had started her menses about 2 months prior to the evaluation. Her family history was pertinent for multiple first- and second-degree relatives with mood, anxiety, or learning disorders.

At first meeting, Daphne was shy and tense. Her eye contact was poor, and she had difficulty talking about anything other than her plastic horse collection. Within 15 minutes, she became more comfortable, revealing that she disliked school because the work was hard and the other children did not seem to care for her. She said that she was afraid of making mistakes and getting bad grades and of disappointing her teachers and parents. Preoccupation with earlier failures led to inattention and indecision. Daphne denied that she was good at anything and that any aspect of her life was going well. She wished she had more friends. As far as she could remember, she had always felt this way. These things made her sad, but she denied persistent depressive feelings or suicidal thoughts. She appeared anxious but brightened when discussing her horse figurine collection and her family.

## Diagnoses

- Specific learning disorder (mathematics)
- Generalized anxiety disorder

## Discussion

Daphne has symptoms of inattention, anxiety, academic difficulties, limited peer relationships, and poor self-esteem that are causing distress and impaired functioning. Biologically, Daphne is experiencing the hormonal changes of puberty against the backdrop of a family history of mood, anxiety, and learning disorders. Psychologically, Daphne is living with the belief that she is inadequate, probably connected with her ongoing difficulties in school. Developmentally, Daphne is functioning at the emotional level of a school-age child. Socially, Daphne has a supportive family environment that has emphasized protecting her, possibly interfering with the acquisition of skills related to independence and autonomy. Meanwhile, the educational system has not provided the necessary support for Daphne to succeed academically.

Daphne's academic problems can be explained in part by a specific learning disorder in mathematics. She has persistent difficulties in this area, supported by testing that showed her performance to be below her intellectual level and chronological age. Her achievement in other academic subjects and her level of adaptive functioning generally appear to be age appropriate, indicating that her global intelligence and adaptive functioning are normal and that she does not have an intellectual disability.

It can be difficult to distinguish between anxiety and mood disorders in children Daphne's age. In this case, an anxiety disorder is more likely because Daphne's symptoms have been chronic rather than episodic, as depressive symptoms often are. Daphne's sadness is related to her sense of failure and worry about her competence. With the exception of a sleep disturbance, she does not have neurovegetative symptoms. Her difficulty with falling asleep sounds anxiety based, as do her social ineptitude, reluctance to comply with school demands, and overreaction when faced with unwelcome tasks. In addition to her anxiety about her capabilities, Daphne appears to have concerns about security, which may explain her tense appearance. Daphne manages her anxieties by avoiding or controlling activities. Although some of her concerns are consistent with other anxiety disorders, such as social anxiety disorder (social phobia) or separation anxiety disorder, Daphne's worries extend beyond those domains. Given the pervasiveness of her anxiety, the most appropriate diagnosis is generalized anxiety disorder (GAD).

GAD is characterized by persistent, excessive anxiety and worry. Symptom criteria include restlessness, poor concentration, irritability, muscle tension, sleep disturbance, and being easily fatigued. Although three of six criteria are required for adults, a GAD diagnosis can be made in children with only one symptom in addition to the excessive anxiety and worry.

Social difficulties are common among children and adolescents, particularly those with psychiatric disorders. Daphne's issues are related to her anxiety about being competent and likable. Her academic struggles and anxiety have impeded her development, making her emotionally and socially immature.

Her immaturity might suggest an autism spectrum disorder. She does have difficulty initiating social interactions and engaging in reciprocity with peers (with poor eye contact notable on examination), but Daphne does not have the communication difficulties, rigidity, or stereotyped behaviors associated with autism. Her behavior improves with familiarity, and she expresses interest in her peers.

Similarly, her language, speech, and communication skills also seem developmentally appropriate, making disorders in these areas unlikely.

Oppositional defiant disorder might also be considered because Daphne is resistant and uncooperative in school and at home when it comes to her academic work. However, this attitude and behavior do not carry over to other situations, and her behaviors do not meet oppositional defiant disorder's requirements for symptom level and frequency. They are better conceptualized as a manifestation of anxiety and an attempt at its management.

Inattention is a symptom that occurs in a variety of diagnoses. Individuals with ADHD have problems with attention, impulsivity, and/or hyperactivity that occur in multiple settings prior to age 12 and cause significant impairment. Although Daphne has several symptoms consistent with inattention, these seem confined to school settings. She also does not appear to have significant problems with behaviors related to impulsivity or activity regulation. ADHD should remain a diagnostic possibility, but other diagnoses better account for Daphne's difficulties.

## Suggested Readings

Connolly SD, Bernstein GA; Work Group on Quality Issues: Practice parameter for the assessment and treatment of children and adolescents with anxiety disorders. J Am Acad Child Adolesc Psychiatry 46(2):267–283, 2007

Lagae L: Learning disabilities: definitions, epidemiology, diagnosis, and intervention strategies. Pediatr Clin North Am 55(6):1259–1268, 2008

# Case 5: Fidgety and Distracted

*Robert Haskell, M.D.*
*John T. Walkup, M.D.*

Ethan, a 9-year-old boy, was referred to a psychiatric clinic by his teacher, who noticed that his attention was flagging. At that time, Ethan was a fourth grader at a private regular-education school for boys. The teacher told Ethan's parents that although Ethan had been among the best students in his class in the fall, his grades had slipped during the spring semester. He tended to get fidgety and distracted when the academic work became more challenging, and the teacher suggested the parents seek neuropsychiatric testing for him.

At home, Ethan's mother explained, he seemed more emotional of late: "He just looks weepy sometimes, which is unusual for him." She denied any difficulties at home, and she described her husband, son, 8-year-old daughter, and herself as a "happy family." She had noticed, however, that Ethan seemed uneasy about being left alone. He had become "clingy," often following his parents around the house, and he hated being in any room by himself. Ethan had also started climbing into bed with his parents in the middle of the night, something he had never done in the past. Although Ethan had a few good friends in the neighborhood and at school and was glad to have other kids come to his house, he refused to go on sleepovers.

Ethan's mother agreed that he appeared more fidgety. She had noticed that he often seemed to be shrugging his shoulders, grimacing, and blinking, which she took to be a sign of anxiety. These movements worsened when he was tired or frustrated, and they diminished in frequency during calm, focused activities such as clarinet practice or homework, especially when she was helping him.

His mother also mentioned that Ethan had suddenly become "superstitious." Whenever he stepped through a doorway, he would go back and forth until he touched both doorjambs with his hands simultaneously, twice in rapid succession. She hoped that Ethan's more conspicuous habits would subside by summer, when the family took its annual vacation. She felt that it was the right year for Disneyland, but Ethan's father had suggested taking him on a fishing trip ("just the boys") while mother and daughter visited relatives in New York City.

Ethan's mother recalled her son as an "easy child, but sensitive." He was the product of a planned, uncomplicated pregnancy and met all his developmental milestones on time. He had no history of medical problems or recent infections, but his mother mentioned that he had begun to make frequent visits to the school nurse's office complaining of stomachaches.

On examination, Ethan was a slightly built boy with fair, freckly skin and blond hair. He was somewhat fidgety, tugging at his pants and shifting in his seat. Hearing his mother talk about his new movements seemed to provoke them, and the examiner noted that Ethan also occasionally blinked tightly, rolled his eyes, and made throat-clearing noises. Ethan said that he sometimes worried about "bad things" happening to his parents. His concerns were vague, however, and he seemed to fear only that burglars might break into their house.

## Diagnoses

- Provisional tic disorder
- Separation anxiety disorder

# Discussion

Ethan presents with declining school performance, which his family seems to attribute to a cluster of anxiety symptoms that are of relatively recent onset. He is uneasy with solitude and reluctant to attend sleepovers, has fears that bad things will happen to his parents, and makes frequent trips to the school nurse. He appears to meet criteria for DSM-5 separation anxiety disorder, the symptoms of which need only persist for 1 month in children and adolescents.

Ethan's mother also points out that he has become more fidgety. She links his shoulder shrugging, grimacing, and blinking to this recent onset of separation anxiety. Neither the parents nor the teacher appears to recognize these movements as tics, which are nonrhythmic movements of short duration and sudden onset. Ethan appears to have a variety of tics, including those observed by the interviewer: some motor (blinks, shoulder rolls) and some vocal (chirps, grunts, throat clearing, sniffs, clicks). Tics can be simple, meaning that they last only milliseconds, or complex, which are of longer duration or consist of a chain or sequence of movements. Although tics may vary broadly throughout the course of a tic disorder, they tend to recur in a specific repertoire during any given period of the illness.

The specific tic disorder (if any) is determined by the type and duration of movements. In Tourette's disorder, both motor and vocal tics must be present, whereas in persistent (chronic) motor or vocal tic disorder, only motor or vocal tics are present. Ethan has a mixture of tics, but at this point they have been present for only about 6 months—not the minimum of 1 year required for either Tourette's disorder or persistent tic disorder. Therefore, Ethan is diagnosed with provisional tic disorder.

Tics occur in 15%–20% of children, and it appears that 0.6%–1.0% develop Tourette's disorder. On average, tics emerge between ages 4 and 6, reach peak severity by age 10–12, and generally decline in severity during adolescence. Tics first observed in adulthood were very likely present but unnoticed in childhood. Tics are typically worsened by anxiety, excitement, and exhaustion and abate during calm, focused activity—which is why that fishing trip with dad may be Ethan's best bet for a summer vacation.

Anxiety likely explains Ethan's inattention in the classroom. Although attention-deficit/hyperactivity disorder, inattentive subtype, cannot be ruled out, it seems more probable that tics and anxiety have taken Ethan off task, as he has no early history of inattention or hyperactivity. His success in the fall semester all but rules out a learning disorder, so no testing is indicated. (As a rule, testing should always follow the treatment of a confounding problem such as anxiety.) As for obsessive-compulsive disorder, an illness associated with both anxiety and tic disorders, Ethan's rituals in the doorway would have to be distressing or impairing before this diagnosis can be entertained.

# Suggested Readings

Plessen KJ: Tic disorders and Tourette's syndrome. Eur Child Adolesc Psychiatry 22 (suppl 1):S55–S60, 2013

Walkup JT, Ferrão Y, Leckman JF, et al: Tic disorders: some key issues for DSM-V. Depress Anxiety 27:600–610, 2010

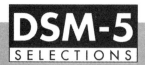

1.  Which of the following is *not* required for a DSM-5 diagnosis of intellectual disability (intellectual developmental disorder)?

    A. Full-scale IQ below 70.
    B. Deficits in intellectual functions confirmed by clinical assessment.
    C. Deficits in adaptive functioning that result in failure to meet developmental and sociocultural standards for personal independence and social responsibility.
    D. Symptom onset during the developmental period.
    E. Deficits in intellectual functions confirmed by individualized, standardized intelligence testing.

2.  A 7-year-old boy in second grade displays significant delays in his ability to reason, solve problems, and learn from his experiences. He has been slow to develop reading, writing, and mathematics skills in school. All through development, these skills lagged behind peers, although he is making slow progress. These deficits significantly impair his ability to play in an age-appropriate manner with peers and to begin to acquire independent skills at home. He requires ongoing assistance with basic skills (dressing, feeding, and bathing himself; doing any type of schoolwork) on a daily basis. Which of the following diagnoses best fits this presentation?

    A. Childhood-onset major neurocognitive disorder.
    B. Specific learning disorder.
    C. Intellectual disability (intellectual developmental disorder).
    D. Communication disorder.
    E. Autism spectrum disorder.

3.  A 7-year-old boy in second grade displays significant delays in his ability to reason, solve problems, and learn from his experiences. He has been slow to develop reading, writing, and mathematics skills in school. All through development, these skills lagged behind peers, although he is making slow progress. These deficits significantly impair his ability to play in an age-appropriate manner with peers and to begin to acquire independent skills at home. He requires ongoing assistance with basic skills (dressing, feeding, and bathing himself; doing any type of schoolwork) on a daily basis. What is the appropriate severity rating for this patient's current presentation?

    A. Mild.
    B. Moderate.
    C. Severe.
    D. Profound.
    E. Cannot be determined without an IQ score.

4. Which of the following statements about intellectual disability (intellectual developmental disorder) is *false?*

    A. Individuals with intellectual disability have deficits in general mental abilities and impairment in everyday adaptive functioning compared with age- and gender-matched peers from the same linguistic and sociocultural group.
    B. For individuals with intellectual disability, the full-scale IQ score is a valid assessment of overall mental abilities and adaptive functioning, even if subtest scores are highly discrepant.
    C. Individuals with intellectual disability may have difficulty in managing their behavior, emotions, and interpersonal relationships and in maintaining motivation in the learning process.
    D. Intellectual disability is generally associated with an IQ that is 2 standard deviations from the population mean, which equates to an IQ score of about 70 or below (±5 points).
    E. Assessment procedures for intellectual disability must take into account factors that may limit performance, such as sociocultural background, native language, associated communication/language disorder, and motor or sensory handicap.

5. Which of the following statements about the diagnosis of intellectual disability (intellectual developmental disorder) is *false?*

    A. An individual with an IQ of less than 70 would receive the diagnosis if there were no significant deficits in adaptive functioning.
    B. An individual with an IQ above 75 would not meet diagnostic criteria even if there were impairments in adaptive functioning.
    C. In forensic assessment, severe deficits in adaptive functioning might allow for a diagnosis with an IQ above 75.
    D. Adaptive functioning must take into account the three domains of conceptual, social, and practical functioning.
    E. The specifiers mild, moderate, severe, and profound are based on IQ scores.

6. Which of the following is *not* a diagnostic feature of intellectual disability (intellectual developmental disorder)?

    A. A full-scale IQ of less than 70.
    B. Inability to perform complex daily living tasks (e.g., money management, medical decision making) without support.
    C. Gullibility, with naiveté in social situations and a tendency to be easily led by others.

   D. Lack of age-appropriate communication skills for social and interpersonal functioning.
   E. All of the above are diagnostic features of intellectual disability.

7. Which of the following statements about adaptive functioning in the diagnosis of intellectual disability (intellectual developmental disorder) is *true?*

   A. Adaptive functioning is based on an individual's IQ score.
   B. "Deficits in adaptive functioning" refers to problems with motor coordination.
   C. At least two domains of adaptive functioning must be impaired to meet Criterion B for the diagnosis of intellectual disability.
   D. Adaptive functioning in intellectual disability tends to improve over time, although the threshold of cognitive capacities and associated developmental disorders can limit it.
   E. Individuals diagnosed with intellectual disability in childhood will typically continue to meet criteria in adulthood even if their adaptive functioning improves.

8. Which of the following statements about development of and risk factors for intellectual disability (intellectual developmental disorder) is *true?*

   A. Intellectual developmental disorder should not be diagnosed in the presence of a known genetic syndrome, such as Lesch-Nyhan or Prader-Willi syndrome.
   B. Etiologies are confined to perinatal and postnatal factors and exclude prenatal events.
   C. In severe acquired forms of intellectual developmental disorder, onset may be abrupt following an illness (e.g., meningitis) or head trauma occurring during the developmental period.
   D. When intellectual disability results from a loss of previously acquired cognitive skills, as in severe traumatic brain injury (TBI), only the TBI diagnosis is assigned.
   E. Prenatal, perinatal, and postnatal etiologies of intellectual developmental disorder are demonstrable in approximately 33% of cases.

9. Which of the following statements about the developmental course of intellectual disability (intellectual developmental disorder) is *true?*

   A. Delayed motor, language, and social milestones are not identifiable until after the first 2 years of life.
   B. Intellectual disability caused by an illness (e.g., encephalitis) or by head trauma occurring during the developmental period would be diagnosed as a neurocognitive disorder, not as intellectual disability (intellectual developmental disorder).
   C. Intellectual disability is always nonprogressive.

    D. Major neurocognitive disorder may co-occur with intellectual developmental disorder.

    E. Even if early and ongoing interventions throughout childhood and adulthood lead to improved adaptive and intellectual functioning, the diagnosis of intellectual disability would continue to apply.

10. The DSM-5 diagnosis of intellectual developmental disorder includes severity specifiers—Mild, Moderate, Severe, and Profound—with which to indicate the level of supports required in various domains of adaptive functioning. Which of the following features would *not* be characteristic of an individual with a "Severe" level of impairment?

    A. The individual generally has little understanding of written language or of concepts involving numbers, quantity, time, and money.

    B. The individual's spoken language is quite limited in terms of vocabulary and grammar.

    C. The individual requires support for all activities of daily living, including meals, dressing, bathing, and toileting.

    D. In adulthood, the individual may be able to sustain competitive employment in a job that does not emphasize conceptual skills.

    E. The individual cannot make responsible decisions regarding the well-being of self or others.

11. A 10-year-old boy with a history of dyslexia, who is otherwise developmentally normal, is in a skateboarding accident in which he experiences severe traumatic brain injury. This results in significant global intellectual impairment (with a persistent reading deficit that is more pronounced than his other newly acquired but stable deficits, along with a full-scale IQ of 75). There is mild impairment in his adaptive functioning such that he requires support in some areas of functioning. He is also displaying anxious and depressive symptoms in response to his accident and hospitalization. What is the *least likely* diagnosis?

    A. Intellectual disability (intellectual developmental disorder).

    B. Traumatic brain injury.

    C. Specific learning disorder.

    D. Major neurocognitive disorder due to traumatic brain injury.

    E. Adjustment disorder.

12. In which of the following situations would a diagnosis of global developmental delay be *inappropriate*?

    A. The patient is a child who is too young to fully manifest specific symptoms or to complete requisite assessments.

    B. The patient, a 7-year-old boy, has a full-scale IQ of 65 and severe impairment in adaptive functioning.

    C. The patient's scores on psychometric tests suggest intellectual disability (intellectual developmental disorder), but there is insufficient information about the patient's adaptive functional skills.

    D. The patient's impaired adaptive functioning suggests intellectual developmental disorder, but there is insufficient information about the level of cognitive impairment measured by standardized instruments.

    E. The patient's cognitive and adaptive impairments suggest intellectual developmental disorder, but there is insufficient information about age at onset of the condition.

13. Which of the following statements about global developmental delay is *true?*

    A. The diagnosis is typically made in children younger than 5 years of age.
    B. The etiology can usually be determined.
    C. The prevalence is estimated to be between 0.5% and 2%.
    D. The condition is progressive.
    E. The condition does not generally occur with other neurodevelopmental disorders.

14. A 3½-year-old girl with a history of lead exposure and a seizure disorder demonstrates substantial delays across multiple domains of functioning, including communication, learning, attention, and motor development, which limit her ability to interact with same-age peers and require substantial support in all activities of daily living at home. Unfortunately, her mother is an extremely poor historian, and the child has received no formal psychological or learning evaluation to date. She is about to be evaluated for readiness to attend preschool. What is the most appropriate diagnosis?

    A. Major neurocognitive disorder.
    B. Developmental coordination disorder.
    C. Autism spectrum disorder.
    D. Global developmental delay.
    E. Specific learning disorder.

15. A 5-year-old boy has difficulty making friends and problems with initiating and sustaining back-and-forth conversation; reading social cues; and sharing his feelings with others. He makes good eye contact, has normal speech intonation, displays facial gestures, and has a range of affect that generally seems appropriate to the situation. He demonstrates an interest in trains that seems abnormal in intensity and focus, and he engages in little imaginative or symbolic play. Which of the following diagnostic requirements for autism spectrum disorder are *not* met in this case?

    A. Deficits in social-emotional reciprocity.
    B. Deficits in nonverbal communicative behaviors used for social interaction.
    C. Deficits in developing and maintaining relationships.
    D. Restricted, repetitive patterns of behavior, interests, or activities as manifested by symptoms in two of the specified four categories.
    E. Symptoms with onset in early childhood that cause clinically significant impairment.

16. Which of the following statements about the development and course of autism spectrum disorder (ASD) is *false?*

    A. Symptoms of ASD are typically recognized during the second year of life (12–24 months of age).
    B. Symptoms of ASD are usually not noticeable until 5–6 years of age or later.
    C. First symptoms frequently involve delayed language development, often accompanied by lack of social interest or unusual social interactions.
    D. ASD is not a degenerative disorder, and it is typical for learning and compensation to continue throughout life.
    E. Because many normally developing young children have strong preferences and enjoy repetition, distinguishing restricted and repetitive behaviors that are diagnostic of ASD can be difficult in preschoolers.

17. Which of the following was a criterion symptom for autistic disorder in DSM-IV that was eliminated from the diagnostic criteria for autism spectrum disorder in DSM-5?

    A. Stereotyped or restricted patterns of interest.
    B. Stereotyped and repetitive motor mannerisms.
    C. Inflexible adherence to routines.
    D. Persistent preoccupation with parts of objects.
    E. None of the above.

18. A 7-year-old girl presents with a history of normal language skills (vocabulary and grammar intact) but is unable to use language in a socially pragmatic manner to share ideas and feelings. She has never made good eye contact, and she has difficulty reading social cues. Consequently, she has had difficulty making friends, which is further complicated by her being somewhat obsessed with cartoon characters, which she repetitively scripts. She tends to excessively smell objects. Because she insists on wearing the same shirt and shorts every day, regardless of the season, getting dressed is a difficult activity. These symptoms date from early childhood and cause significant impairment in her functioning. What diagnosis best fits this child's presentation?

    A. Asperger's disorder.
    B. Autism spectrum disorder.
    C. Pervasive developmental disorder not otherwise specified (NOS).
    D. Social (pragmatic) communication disorder.
    E. Rett syndrome.

19. A 15-year-old boy has a long history of nonverbal communication deficits. As an infant he was unable to follow someone else directing his attention by pointing. As a toddler he was not interested in sharing events, feelings, or games with his parents. From school age into adolescence, his speech was odd in tonality and phrasing, and his body language was awkward. What do these symptoms represent?

    A. Stereotypies.

    B. Restricted range of interests.

    C. Developmental regression.

    D. Prodromal schizophreniform symptoms.

    E. Deficits in nonverbal communicative behaviors.

20. A 10-year-old boy demonstrates hand-flapping and finger flicking, and he repetitively flips coins and lines up his trucks. He tends to "echo" the last several words of a question posed to him before answering, mixes up his pronouns (refers to himself in the second person), tends to repeat phrases in a perseverative fashion, and is quite fixated on routines related to dress, eating, travel, and play. He spends hours in his garage playing with his father's tools. What do these behaviors represent?

    A. Restricted, repetitive patterns of behaviors, interests, or activities characteristic of autism spectrum disorder.

    B. Symptoms of obsessive-compulsive disorder.

    C. Prototypical manifestations of obsessive-compulsive personality.

    D. Symptoms of pediatric acute-onset neuropsychiatric syndrome (PANS).

    E. Complex tics.

21. A 25-year-old man presents with long-standing nonverbal communication deficits, inability to have a back-and-forth conversation or share interests in an appropriate fashion, and a complete lack of interest in having relationships with others. His speech reflects awkward phrasing and intonation and is mechanical in nature. He has a history of sequential fixations and obsessions with various games and objects throughout childhood; however, this is not currently a major issue for him. This patient meets criteria for autism spectrum disorder; true or false?

    A. True.

    B. False.

22. A 9-year-old girl presents with a history of intellectual impairment, a structural language impairment, nonverbal communication deficits, disinterest in peers, and inability to use language in a social manner. She has extreme food and tactile sensitivities. She is obsessed with one particular computer game that she plays for hours each day, and she scripts and imitates the characters in this game. She is clumsy, has an odd gait, and walks on her tiptoes. In the past year she has developed a seizure disorder and has begun to bang her wrists against the wall repetitively, causing bruising. On the other hand, she plays several musical instruments in an extremely precocious manner. Which feature of this child's clinical presentation fulfills a criterion symptom for DSM-5 autism spectrum disorder?

    A. Motor abnormalities.

    B. Seizures.

    C. Structural language impairment.

    D. Intellectual impairment.

    E. Nonverbal communicative deficits.

23. An 11-year-old girl with autism spectrum disorder displays no spoken language and is minimally responsive to overtures from others. She can be somewhat inflexible, which interferes with her ability to travel, do schoolwork, and be managed in the home; she has some difficulty transitioning; and she has trouble organizing and planning activities. These problems can usually be managed with incentives and reinforcers. What severity levels should be specified in the DSM-5 diagnosis?

    A. Level 3 (requiring very substantial support) for social communication, and level 1 (requiring support) for restricted, repetitive behaviors.

    B. Level 1 (requiring support) for social communication, and level 3 (requiring very substantial support) for restricted, repetitive behaviors.

    C. Level 1 (requiring support) for social communication, and level 2 (requiring substantial support) for restricted, repetitive behaviors.

    D. Level 3 (requiring very substantial support) for social communication, and level 1 (requiring support) for restricted, repetitive behaviors.

    E. Level 2 (requiring substantial support) for social communication, and level 1 (requiring support) for restricted, repetitive behaviors.

24. Which of the following is *not* a specifier included in the diagnostic criteria for autism spectrum disorder?

    A. With or without accompanying intellectual impairment.

    B. With or without associated dementia.

    C. With or without accompanying language impairment.

    D. Associated with a known medical or genetic condition or environmental factor.

    E. Associated with another neurodevelopmental, mental, or behavioral disorder.

25. Which of the following is *not* characteristic of the developmental course of children diagnosed with autism spectrum disorder?

    A. Behavioral features manifest before 3 years of age.

    B. The full symptom pattern does not appear until age 2–3 years.

    C. Developmental plateaus or regression in social-communicative behavior is frequently reported by parents.

    D. Regression across multiple domains occurs after age 2–3 years.

    E. First symptoms often include delayed language development, lack of social interest or unusual social behavior, odd play, and unusual communication patterns.

26. A 5-year-old girl has some mild food aversions. She enjoys having the same book read to her at night but does not become terribly upset if her mother asks her to choose a different book. She occasionally spins around excitedly when her favorite show is on. She generally likes her toys neatly arranged in bins but is only mildly upset when her sister leaves them on the floor. These behaviors should be considered suspicious for an autism spectrum disorder; true or false?

    A. True.
    B. False.

27. Which of the following is *not* representative of the typical developmental course for autism spectrum disorder?

    A. Lack of degenerative course.
    B. Behavioral deterioration during adolescence.
    C. Continued learning and compensation throughout life.
    D. Marked presence of symptoms in early childhood and early school years, with developmental gains in later childhood in areas such as social interaction.
    E. Good psychosocial functioning in adulthood, as indexed by independent living and gainful employment.

28. A 21-year-old man, not previously diagnosed with a developmental disorder, presents for evaluation after taking a leave from college for psychological reasons. He makes little eye contact, does not appear to pick up on social cues, has become disinterested in friends, spends hours each day on the computer surfing the Internet and playing games, and has become so sensitive to smells that he keeps multiple air fresheners in all locations of the home. He reports that he has had long-standing friendships dating from childhood and high school (corroborated by his parents). He reports making many friends in his fraternity at college. His parents report good social and communication skills in childhood, although he was quite shy and was somewhat inflexible and ritualistic at home. What is the *least likely* diagnosis?

    A. Depression.
    B. Schizophreniform disorder or schizophrenia.
    C. Autism spectrum disorder.
    D. Obsessive-compulsive disorder.
    E. Social anxiety disorder (social phobia).

29. Which of the following characteristics is generally *not* associated with autism spectrum disorder?

    A. Anxiety, depression, and isolation as an adult.
    B. Catatonia.
    C. Poor psychosocial functioning.
    D. Insistence on routines and aversion to change.
    E. Successful adaptation in regular school settings.

30. Which of the following disorders is generally *not* comorbid with autism spectrum disorder (ASD)?

    A. Attention-deficit/hyperactivity disorder (ADHD).
    B. Rett syndrome.
    C. Selective mutism.
    D. Intellectual disability (intellectual developmental disorder).
    E. Stereotypic movement disorder.

31. Which of the following is *not* a criterion for the DSM-5 diagnosis of attention-deficit/hyperactivity disorder (ADHD)?

    A. Onset of several inattentive or hyperactive-impulsive symptoms prior to age 12 years.
    B. Manifestation of several inattentive or hyperactive-impulsive symptoms in two or more settings (e.g., at home, school, or work; with friends or relatives; in other activities).
    C. Persistence of symptoms for at least 12 months.
    D. Clear evidence that symptoms interfere with, or reduce the quality of, social, academic, or occupational functioning.
    E. Inability to explain symptoms as a manifestation of another mental disorder (e.g., mood disorder, anxiety disorder, dissociative disorder, personality disorder, substance intoxication or withdrawal).

32. The parents of a 15-year-old female tenth grader believe that she should be doing better in high school, given how bright she seems and the fact that she received mostly A's through eighth grade. Her papers are handed in late, and she makes careless mistakes on examinations. They have her tested, and the WAIS-IV results are as follows: Verbal IQ, 125; Perceptual Reasoning Index, 122; Full-Scale IQ, 123; Working Memory Index, 55th percentile; Processing Speed Index, 50th percentile. Weaknesses in executive function are noted. During a psychiatric evaluation, she reports a long history of failing to give close attention to details, difficulty sustaining attention while in class or doing homework, failing to finish chores and tasks, and significant difficulties with time management, planning, and organization. She is forgetful, often loses things, and is easily distracted. She has no history of restlessness or impulsivity, and she is well liked by her peers. What is the most likely diagnosis?

    A. Adjustment disorder with anxiety.
    B. Specific learning disorder.
    C. Attention-deficit/hyperactivity disorder, predominantly inattentive.
    D. Developmental coordination disorder.
    E. Major depressive disorder.

33. A 7-year-old boy is having behavioral and social difficulties in his second-grade class. Although he seems to be able to attend and is doing "well" from an academic standpoint (though seemingly not what he is capable of), he is

constantly interrupting, fidgeting, talking excessively, and getting out of his seat. He has friends, but he sometimes annoys his peers because of his difficulty sharing and taking turns and the fact that he is constantly talking over them. Although he seeks out play dates, his friends tire of him because he wants to play sports nonstop. At home, he can barely stay in his seat for a meal and is unable to play quietly. Although he shows remorse when the consequences of his behavior are pointed out to him, he can become angry in response and seems nevertheless unable to inhibit himself. What is the most likely diagnosis?

A. Bipolar disorder.
B. Autism spectrum disorder.
C. Generalized anxiety disorder.
D. Attention-deficit/hyperactivity disorder, predominantly hyperactive/impulsive.
E. Specific learning disorder.

34. A 37-year-old Wall Street trader schedules a visit after his 8-year-old son is diagnosed with attention-deficit/hyperactivity disorder (ADHD), combined inattentive and hyperactive. Although he does not currently note motor restlessness like his son, he recalls being that way when he was a boy, along with being quite inattentive, being impulsive, talking excessively, interrupting, and having problems waiting his turn. He was an underachiever in high school and college, when he inconsistently did his work and had difficulty following rules. Nevertheless, he never failed any classes, and he was never evaluated by a psychologist or psychiatrist. He works about 60–80 hours a week and often gets insufficient sleep. He tends to make impulsive business decisions, can be impatient and short-tempered, and notes that his mind tends to wander both in one-on-one interactions with associates and his wife and during business meetings, for which he is often late; he is forgetful and disorganized. Nevertheless, he tends to perform fairly well and is quite successful, although he can occasionally feel overwhelmed and demoralized. What is the most likely diagnosis?

A. Major depressive disorder.
B. Generalized anxiety disorder.
C. Specific learning disorder.
D. ADHD, in partial remission.
E. Oppositional defiant disorder.

35. A 5-year-old hyperactive, impulsive, and inattentive boy presents with hypertelorism, highly arched palate, and low-set ears. He is uncoordinated and clumsy, he has no sense of time, and his toys and clothes are constantly strewn all over the house. He has recently developed what appears to be a motor tic involving blinking. He enjoys playing with peers, who tend to like him, although he seems to willfully defy all requests from his parents and kindergarten teacher, which does not seem to be due simply to inattention. He is delayed in beginning to learn how to read. What is the *least likely* diagnosis?

    A. Autism spectrum disorder.

    B. Developmental coordination disorder.

    C. Oppositional defiant disorder (ODD).

    D. Specific learning disorder.

    E. Attention-deficit/hyperactivity disorder (ADHD).

36. What is the prevalence of attention-deficit/hyperactivity disorder (ADHD) in children?

    A. 8%.

    B. 10%.

    C. 2%.

    D. 0.5%.

    E. 5%.

37. What is the prevalence of attention-deficit/hyperactivity disorder (ADHD) in adults?

    A. 8%.

    B. 10%.

    C. 2.5%.

    D. 0.5%.

    E. 5%.

38. What is the gender ratio of attention-deficit/hyperactivity disorder (ADHD) in children?

    A. Male:female ratio of 2:1.

    B. Male:female ratio of 1:1.

    C. Male:female ratio of 3:2.

    D. Male:female ratio of 5:1.

    E. Male:female ratio of 1:2.

39. Which of the following is a biological finding in individuals with attention-deficit/hyperactivity disorder (ADHD)?

    A. Decreased slow-wave activity on electroencephalograms.

    B. Reduced total brain volume on magnetic resonance imaging.

    C. Early posterior to anterior cortical maturation.

    D. Reduced thalamic volume.

    E. Both B and C.

40. Which of the following is *not* associated with attention-deficit/hyperactivity disorder (ADHD)?

    A. Reduced school performance.

    B. Poorer occupational performance and attendance.

    C. Higher probability of unemployment.

    D. Elevated interpersonal conflict.

    E. Reduced risk of substance use disorders.

41. Which of the following is *not* associated with attention-deficit/hyperactivity disorder (ADHD)?

    A. Social rejection.

    B. Increased risk of developing conduct disorder in childhood and antisocial personality disorder in adulthood.

    C. Increased risk of Alzheimer's disease.

    D. Increased frequency of traffic accidents and violations.

    E. Increased risk of accidental injury.

42. A 15-year-old boy has developed concentration problems in school that have been associated with a significant decline in grades. When interviewed, he explains that his mind is occupied with worrying about his mother, who has a serious autoimmune disease. As his grades falter, he becomes increasingly demoralized and sad, and he notices that his energy level drops, further compromising his ability to pay attention in school. At the same time, he complains of feeling restless and unable to sleep. What is the most likely diagnosis?

    A. Bipolar disorder.

    B. Specific learning disorder.

    C. Attention-deficit/hyperactivity disorder (ADHD).

    D. Adjustment disorder with mixed anxiety and depressed mood.

    E. Separation anxiety disorder.

43. A 5-year-old boy is consistently moody, irritable, and intolerant of frustration. In addition, he is pervasively and chronically restless, impulsive, and inattentive. Which diagnosis best fits his clinical picture?

    A. Attention-deficit/hyperactivity disorder (ADHD).

    B. ADHD and disruptive mood dysregulation disorder (DMDD).

    C. Bipolar disorder.

    D. Oppositional defiant disorder (ODD).

    E. Major depressive disorder (MDD).

44. Which of the following statements about comorbidity in attention-deficit/hyperactivity disorder (ADHD) is *true?*

    A. Oppositional defiant disorder co-occurs with ADHD in about half of children with the combined presentation and about a quarter of those with the predominantly inattentive presentation.

    B. Most children with disruptive mood dysregulation disorder do not also meet criteria for ADHD.

    C. Fifteen percent of adults with ADHD have some type of anxiety disorder.

    D. Intermittent explosive disorder occurs in about 5% of adults with ADHD.

    E. Specific learning disorder very seldom co-occurs with ADHD.

45. Specific learning disorder is defined by persistent difficulties in learning academic skills, with onset during the developmental period. Which of the following statements about this disorder is *true?*

    A. It is part of a more general learning impairment as manifested in intellectual disability (intellectual developmental disorder).
    B. It can usually be attributed to a sensory, physical, or neurological disorder.
    C. It involves pervasive and wide-ranging deficits across multiple domains of information processing.
    D. It can be caused by external factors such as economic disadvantage or lack of education.
    E. It replaces the DSM-IV diagnoses of reading disorder, mathematics disorder, disorder of written expression, and learning disorder not otherwise specified.

46. In distinction to DSM-IV, DSM-5 classifies all learning disorders under the diagnosis of specific learning disorder, along with the requirement to "specify all academic domains and subskills that are impaired" at the time of assessment. Which of the following statements about specific learning disorder is *false?*

    A. There are persistent difficulties in the acquisition of reading, writing, arithmetic, or mathematical reasoning skills during the formal years of schooling.
    B. Current skills in one or more of these academic areas are well below the average range for the individual's age, gender, cultural group, and level of education.
    C. There usually is a discrepancy of more than 2 standard deviations (SD) between achievement and IQ.
    D. The learning difficulties significantly interfere with academic achievement, occupational performance, or activities of daily living that require these academic skills.
    E. The learning difficulties cannot be acquired later in life.

47. Which of the following statements about the diagnosis of specific learning disorder is *false?*

    A. Specific learning disorder is distinct from learning problems associated with a neurodegenerative cognitive disorder.
    B. If intellectual disability (intellectual developmental disorder) is present, the learning difficulties must be in excess of those expected.
    C. An uneven profile of abilities is typical in specific learning disorder.
    D. Attentional difficulties and motor clumsiness that are subthreshold for attention-deficit/hyperactivity disorder or developmental coordination disorder are frequently associated with specific learning disorder.
    E. There are four formal subtypes of specific learning disorder.

48. Which of the following statements about prevalence rates for specific learning disorder is *false?*

    A. Prevalence rates range from 5% to 15% among school-age children across languages and cultures.
    B. Prevalence in adults is approximately 4%.
    C. Specific learning disorder is equally common among males and females.
    D. Prevalence rates vary according to the range of ages in the sample, selection criteria, severity of specific learning disorder, and academic domains investigated.
    E. Gender ratios cannot be attributed to factors such as ascertainment bias, definitional or measurement variation, language, race, or socioeconomic status.

49. Which of the following statements about comorbidity in specific learning disorder is *true?*

    A. Attention-deficit/hyperactivity disorder (ADHD) does not co-occur with specific learning disorder more frequently than would be expected by chance.
    B. Speech sound disorder and specific language impairments are not commonly comorbid with specific learning disorder.
    C. Identified clusters of co-occurrences include severe reading disorders; fine motor problems and handwriting problems; and problems with arithmetic, reading, and gross motor planning.
    D. The co-occurrence of specific learning disorder and specific language impairments has been shown in up to 20% of children with language problems.
    E. Co-occurring disorders generally do not influence the course or treatment of specific learning disorder.

50. Which of the following statements about developmental coordination disorder (DCD) is *true?*

    A. Some children with DCD show additional (usually suppressed) motor activity, such as choreiform movements of unsupported limbs or mirror movements.
    B. The prevalence of DCD in children ages 5–11 years is 1%–3%.
    C. In early adulthood, there is improvement in learning new tasks involving complex/automatic motor skills, including driving and using tools.
    D. DCD has no association with prenatal exposure to alcohol or with low birth weight or preterm birth.
    E. Impairments in underlying neurodevelopmental processes have not been found to primarily affect visuomotor skills.

51. Which of the following statements about developmental coordination disorder (DCD) is *true?*

    A. The disorder is usually not diagnosed before the age of 7 years.
    B. Symptoms have usually improved significantly at 1-year follow-up.
    C. In most cases, symptoms are no longer evident by adolescence.
    D. DCD has no clear relationship with prenatal alcohol exposure, preterm birth, or low birth weight.
    E. Cerebellar dysfunction is hypothesized to play a role in DCD.

52. Which of the following is *not* a criterion for the DSM-5 diagnosis of stereotypic movement disorder?

    A. Motor behaviors are present that are repetitive, seemingly driven, and apparently purposeless.
    B. Onset of the behaviors is in the early developmental period.
    C. The behaviors result in self-inflicted bodily injury that requires medical treatment.
    D. The behaviors are not attributable to the physiological effects of a substance or neurological condition or better explained by another neurodevelopmental or mental disorder.
    E. The behaviors interfere with social, academic, or other activities.

53. Which of the following statements about the developmental course of stereotypic movement disorder is *false?*

    A. The presence of stereotypic movements may indicate an undetected neurodevelopmental problem, especially in children ages 1–3 years.
    B. Among typically developing children, the repetitive movements may be stopped when attention is directed to them or when the child is distracted from performing them.
    C. In some children, the stereotypic movements would result in self-injury if protective measures were not used.
    D. Whereas simple stereotypic movements (e.g., rocking) are common in young typically developing children, complex stereotypic movements are much less common (approximately 3%–4%).
    E. Stereotypic movements typically begin within the first year of life.

54. Which of the following is a DSM-5 diagnostic criterion for Tourette's disorder?

    A. Tics occur throughout a period of more than 1 year, and during this period there was never a tic-free period of more than 3 consecutive months.
    B. Onset is before age 5 years.
    C. The tics may wax and wane in frequency but have persisted for more than 1 year since first tic onset.
    D. Motor tics must precede vocal tics.

    E.  The tics may occur many times a day for at least 4 weeks, but no longer than 12 consecutive months.

55.  At her child's third office visit, the mother of an 8-year-old boy with a 6-month history of excessive eye blinking and intermittent chirping says that she has noticed the development of grunting sounds since he started school this term. What is the most likely diagnosis?

    A.  Tourette's disorder.
    B.  Provisional tic disorder.
    C.  Temporary tic disorder.
    D.  Persistent (chronic) vocal tic disorder.
    E.  Transient tic disorder, recurrent.

56.  A 5-year-old girl is referred to your care with a DSM-IV diagnosis of chronic motor or vocal tic disorder. Under DSM-5, she would meet criteria for persistent (chronic) motor or vocal tic disorder. Which of the following statements about her new diagnosis under DSM-5 is *false?*

    A.  She may have single or multiple motor or vocal tics, but not both.
    B.  Her tics must persist for more than 1 year since first tic onset without a tic-free period for 3 consecutive months to meet diagnostic criteria.
    C.  Her tics may wax and wane in frequency but have persisted for more than 1 year since first tic onset.
    D.  She has never met criteria for Tourette's disorder.
    E.  A specifier may be added to the diagnosis of persistent (chronic) motor or vocal tic disorder to indicate whether the girl has motor or vocal tics.

57.  A highly functional 20-year-old college student with a history of anxiety symptoms and attention-deficit/hyperactivity disorder, for which she is prescribed lisdexamfetamine (Vyvanse), tells her psychiatrist that she has been researching the side effects of her medication for one of her class projects. In addition, she says that for the past week she has been feeling stressed by her schoolwork, and her friends have been asking her why she intermittently bobs her head up and down multiple times a day. What is the most likely diagnosis?

    A.  Provisional tic disorder.
    B.  Unspecified tic disorder.
    C.  Unspecified anxiety disorder.
    D.  Obsessive-compulsive personality disorder.
    E.  Unspecified stimulant-induced disorder.

58.  Which of the following is *not* a DSM-5 diagnostic criterion for language disorder?

    A.  Persistent difficulties in the acquisition and use of language across modalities due to deficits in comprehension or production.
    B.  Language abilities that are substantially and quantifiably below those expected for age.

C. Symptom onset in the early developmental period.

D. Inability to attribute difficulties to hearing or other sensory impairment, motor dysfunction, or another medical or neurological condition.

E. Failure to meet criteria for mixed receptive-expressive language disorder or a pervasive developmental disorder.

59. Which of the following statements about speech sound disorder is *true?*

A. Speech sound production must be present by age 2 years.

B. "Failure to use developmentally expected speech sounds" is assessed by comparison of a child with his or her peers of the same age and dialect.

C. The difficulties in speech sound production need not result in functional impairment to meet diagnostic criteria.

D. Symptom onset is in the early developmental period.

E. Both A and C are true.

60. A mother brings her 4-year-old son to you for an evaluation with concerns that her son has struggled with speech articulation since very young. He has not sustained any head injuries, is otherwise healthy, and has a normal IQ. His preschool teacher reports that she does not always understand what he is saying and that other children tease him by calling him a "baby" due to his difficulty with communication. He does not have trouble relating to other people or understanding nonverbal social cues. What is the most likely diagnosis?

A. Selective mutism.

B. Global developmental delay.

C. Speech sound disorder.

D. Avoidant personality disorder.

E. Unspecified anxiety disorder.

61. A 6-year-old boy is failing school and continues to struggle significantly with grammar, sentence construction, and vocabulary. When he speaks, he also interjects "and" in between all his words. His teacher reports that he requires more verbal redirection than other students in order to stay on task. He is generally quiet and does not cause trouble otherwise. Which of the following diagnoses would be on your differential?

A. Language disorder.

B. Expressive language disorder.

C. Childhood-onset fluency disorder.

D. Attention-deficit/hyperactivity disorder (ADHD).

E. A and D.

62. Which of the following types of disturbance in normal speech fluency/time patterning included in the DSM-IV criteria for stuttering was omitted in the DSM-5 criteria for childhood-onset fluency disorder (stuttering)?

A. Sound prolongation.

B. Circumlocution.

C. Interjections.

D. Words produced with an excess of physical tension.

E. Sound and syllable repetitions.

63. A 14-year-old boy in regular education tells you that he thinks a girl in class likes him. His mother is surprised to hear this, because she reports that, since a young age, he has often struggled with making inferences or understanding nuances from what other people say. The teacher has also noticed that he sometimes misses nonverbal cues. He tends to get along better with adults, perhaps because they are not as likely to be put off by his overly formal speech. When he makes jokes, his peers do not always find the humor appropriate. Although he enjoys spending time with his best friend, he can be talkative and struggles with taking turns in conversation. What is the most likely diagnosis?

A. Social (pragmatic) communication disorder.

B. Asperger's disorder.

C. Autism spectrum disorder.

D. Social anxiety disorder.

E. Language disorder.

64. A 15-year-old boy with a prior diagnosis of Tourette's disorder is referred to your care. His mother tells you that during middle school he was teased for having vocal and motor tics. Since starting ninth grade, his tics have become less frequent. Currently, only mild motor tics remain. What is the appropriate DSM-5 diagnosis?

A. Tourette's disorder.

B. Persistent (chronic) motor tic disorder.

C. Provisional tic disorder.

D. Unspecified tic disorder.

E. Persistent (chronic) vocal tic disorder.

65. Tics typically present for the first time during which developmental stage?

A. Infancy.

B. Prepuberty.

C. Latency.

D. Adolescence.

E. Adulthood.

66. A 7-year-old boy who has speech delays presents with long-standing, repetitive hand waving, arm flapping, and finger wiggling. His mother reports that she first noticed these symptoms when he was a toddler and wonders whether they are tics. She says that he tends to flap more when he is engrossed in activities, such as while watching his favorite television program, but will stop when

called or distracted. Based on the mother's report, which of the following conditions would be highest on your list of possible diagnoses?

A. Provisional tic disorder.
B. Persistent (chronic) motor or vocal tic disorder.
C. Chorea.
D. Dystonia.
E. Motor stereotypies.

67. Assessment of co-occurring conditions is important for understanding the overall functional consequence of tics on an individual. Which of the following conditions has been associated with tic disorders?

A. Attention-deficit/hyperactivity disorder (ADHD).
B. Obsessive-compulsive and related disorders.
C. Other movement disorders.
D. Depressive disorders.
E. All of the above.

68. By what age should most children have acquired adequate speech and language ability to understand and follow social rules of verbal and nonverbal communication, follow rules for conversation and storytelling, and change language according to the needs of the listener or situation?

A. Ages 2–3 years.
B. Ages 3–4 years.
C. Ages 4–5 years.
D. Ages 5–6 years.
E. Ages 6–7 years.

69. Having a family history of which of the following psychiatric disorders increases an individual's risk of social (pragmatic) communication disorder?

A. Social anxiety disorder (social phobia).
B. Autism spectrum disorder.
C. Attention-deficit/hyperactivity disorder (ADHD).
D. Specific learning disorder.
E. Either B or D.

70. A 6-year-old boy with a history of mild language delay is brought to your office by his mother, who is concerned that he is being teased in school because he misinterprets nonverbal cues and speaks in overly formal language with his peers. She tells you that her son was in an early intervention program, but his written and spoken language is now at grade level. The boy does not have a history of repetitive movements, sensory issues, or ritualized behaviors. Although he prefers constancy, he adapts fairly well to new situations. Additionally, he has a long-standing interest in trains and cars and is able to recite for

you all the car models he memorized from a book on the history of transportation. Which of the following disorders would be a primary consideration in the differential diagnosis?

A. Social (pragmatic) communication disorder.
B. Autism spectrum disorder.
C. Global developmental delay.
D. Language disorder.
E. A and B.

71. Below what age is it difficult to distinguish a language disorder from normal developmental variations?

A. Age 2 years.
B. Age 3 years.
C. Age 4 years.
D. Age 5 years.
E. Age 6 years.

72. Which of the following psychiatric diagnoses is strongly associated with language disorder?

A. Attention-deficit/hyperactivity disorder.
B. Developmental coordination disorder.
C. Autism spectrum disorder.
D. Social (pragmatic) communication disorder.
E. All of the above.

73. Which of the following statements about the development of speech as it applies to speech sound disorder is *false?*

A. Most children with speech sound disorder respond well to treatment.
B. Speech sound production should be mostly intelligible by age 3 years.
C. Most speech sounds should be pronounced clearly and accurately according to age and community norms before age 10 years.
D. Lisping may or may not be associated with speech sound disorder.
E. It is abnormal for children to shorten words when they are learning to talk.

74. Which of the following would likely *not* be an important condition to rule out in the differential diagnosis of speech sound disorder?

A. Normal variations in speech.
B. Hearing or other sensory impairment.
C. Dysarthria.
D. Depression.
E. Selective mutism.

75. Which of the following statements about the development of childhood-onset fluency disorder (stuttering) is *true?*

    A. Stuttering occurs by age 6 for 80%–90% of affected individuals.
    B. Stuttering always begin abruptly and is noticeable to everyone.
    C. Stress and anxiety do not exacerbate disfluency.
    D. Motor movements are not associated with this disorder.
    E. None of the above.

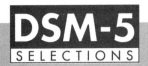

# Neurodevelopmental Disorders

## DSM-5® Self-Exam Answer Guide

1. Which of the following is *not* required for a DSM-5 diagnosis of intellectual disability (intellectual developmental disorder)?

   A. Full-scale IQ below 70.
   B. Deficits in intellectual functions confirmed by clinical assessment.
   C. Deficits in adaptive functioning that result in failure to meet developmental and sociocultural standards for personal independence and social responsibility.
   D. Symptom onset during the developmental period.
   E. Deficits in intellectual functions confirmed by individualized, standardized intelligence testing.

   **Correct Answer: A. Full-scale IQ below 70.**

   **Explanation:** The essential features of intellectual disability (intellectual developmental disorder) relate to both intellectual impairment and deficits in adaptive function. In contrast to DSM-IV, which specified "an IQ of approximately 70 or below" for the former diagnosis of "mental retardation," DSM-5 has no specific requirement for IQ in the renamed diagnosis of intellectual disability.

   1—Intellectual Disability (Intellectual Developmental Disorder) diagnostic criteria (p. 33); Diagnostic Features (p. 37)

2. A 7-year-old boy in second grade displays significant delays in his ability to reason, solve problems, and learn from his experiences. He has been slow to develop reading, writing, and mathematics skills in school. All through development, these skills lagged behind peers, although he is making slow progress. These deficits significantly impair his ability to play in an age-appropriate manner with peers and to begin to acquire independent skills at home. He requires ongoing assistance with basic skills (dressing, feeding, and bathing himself; doing any type of schoolwork) on a daily basis. Which of the following diagnoses best fits this presentation?

   A. Childhood-onset major neurocognitive disorder.
   B. Specific learning disorder.
   C. Intellectual disability (intellectual developmental disorder).
   D. Communication disorder.
   E. Autism spectrum disorder.

**Correct Answer: C. Intellectual disability (intellectual developmental disorder).**

**Explanation:** Intellectual disability is characterized by deficits in general mental abilities, which result in impairments of intellectual and adaptive functioning. In specific learning disorder and communication disorders, there is no general intellectual impairment. Autism spectrum disorder must include history suggesting "persistent deficits in social communication and social interaction across multiple contexts" (Criterion A) or "restricted, repetitive patterns of behavior, interests, or activities" (Criterion B). Intellectual disability is categorized as a neurodevelopmental disorder and is distinct from the neurocognitive disorders, which are characterized by a *loss* of cognitive functioning. There is no evidence for a neurocognitive disorder in this case, although major neurocognitive disorder may co-occur with intellectual disability (e.g., an individual with Down syndrome who develops Alzheimer's disease, or an individual with intellectual disability who loses further cognitive capacity following a head injury). In such cases, the diagnoses of intellectual disability and neurocognitive disorder may both be given.

2—Intellectual Disability (Intellectual Developmental Disorder) / Differential Diagnosis (pp. 39–40)

3. A 7-year-old boy in second grade displays significant delays in his ability to reason, solve problems, and learn from his experiences. He has been slow to develop reading, writing, and mathematics skills in school. All through development, these skills lagged behind peers, although he is making slow progress. These deficits significantly impair his ability to play in an age-appropriate manner with peers and to begin to acquire independent skills at home. He requires ongoing assistance with basic skills (dressing, feeding, and bathing himself; doing any type of schoolwork) on a daily basis. What is the appropriate severity rating for this patient's current presentation?

   A. Mild.
   B. Moderate.
   C. Severe.
   D. Profound.
   E. Cannot be determined without an IQ score.

**Correct Answer: B. Moderate.**

**Explanation:** With respect to severity, the "moderate" qualifier reflects this patient's skills (which have chronically lagged behind those of peers) and his need for assistance in most activities of daily living; however, it also takes into account the fact that he is slowly developing these skills (which would peak at roughly the elementary school level, according to DSM-5).

Although IQ testing would be informative in diagnosing intellectual disability (in previous DSM classifications, subtypes of mild, moderate, severe, and profound were categories based on IQ scores), DSM-5 specifies that *"the various levels of severity are defined on the basis of adaptive functioning, and not IQ scores, because it is adaptive functioning that determines the level of supports required"* (p. 33). Deficits in adaptive functioning refer to how well a person meets community standards of personal independence and social responsibility, in comparison to others of similar age and sociocultural background. Adaptive functioning is assessed using both clinical evaluation and individualized, culturally appropriate, psychometrically sound measures.

Adaptive functioning involves adaptive reasoning in three domains: conceptual, social, and practical. The *conceptual (academic) domain* involves competence in memory, language, reading, writing, math reasoning, acquisition of practical knowledge, problem solving, and judgment in novel situations, among others. The *social domain* involves awareness of others' thoughts, feelings, and experiences; empathy; interpersonal communication skills; friendship abilities; and social judgment, among others. The *practical domain* involves learning and self-management across life settings, including personal care, job responsibilities, money management, recreation, self-management of behavior, and school and work task organization, among others. Intellectual capacity, education, motivation, socialization, personality features, vocational opportunity, cultural experience, and coexisting general medical conditions or mental disorders influence adaptive functioning.

**3—Intellectual Disability (Intellectual Developmental Disorder) / Diagnostic Features (p. 37)**

4. Which of the following statements about intellectual disability (intellectual developmental disorder) is *false?*

   A. Individuals with intellectual disability have deficits in general mental abilities and impairment in everyday adaptive functioning compared with age- and gender-matched peers from the same linguistic and sociocultural group.
   B. For individuals with intellectual disability, the full-scale IQ score is a valid assessment of overall mental abilities and adaptive functioning, even if subtest scores are highly discrepant.
   C. Individuals with intellectual disability may have difficulty in managing their behavior, emotions, and interpersonal relationships and in maintaining motivation in the learning process.
   D. Intellectual disability is generally associated with an IQ that is 2 standard deviations from the population mean, which equates to an IQ score of about 70 or below (±5 points).
   E. Assessment procedures for intellectual disability must take into account factors that may limit performance, such as sociocultural background, native language, associated communication/language disorder, and motor or sensory handicap.

**Correct Answer: B. For individuals with intellectual disability, the full-scale IQ score is a valid assessment of overall mental abilities and adaptive functioning, even if subtest scores are highly discrepant.**

**Explanation:** The single IQ score is an approximation of conceptual functioning, but insufficient alone for assessing mastery of practical tasks and reasoning in real-life situations. Highly discrepant individual subtest scores may make an overall IQ score invalid. Thus, the profile of weaknesses on subtest scores is generally a more accurate reflection of an individual's overall mental abilities than the full-scale IQ.

**4—Intellectual Disability (Intellectual Developmental Disorder) / Diagnostic Features (p. 37)**

5. Which of the following statements about the diagnosis of intellectual disability (intellectual developmental disorder) is *false?*

   A. An individual with an IQ of less than 70 would receive the diagnosis if there were no significant deficits in adaptive functioning.
   B. An individual with an IQ above 75 would not meet diagnostic criteria even if there were impairments in adaptive functioning.
   C. In forensic assessment, severe deficits in adaptive functioning might allow for a diagnosis with an IQ above 75.
   D. Adaptive functioning must take into account the three domains of conceptual, social, and practical functioning.
   E. The specifiers mild, moderate, severe, and profound are based on IQ scores.

**Correct Answer: E. The specifiers mild, moderate, severe, and profound are based on IQ scores.**

**Explanation:** Severity specifiers are included in the diagnostic criteria for intellectual disability (intellectual developmental disorder). The various levels of severity are defined on the basis of adaptive functioning, and not IQ scores, because it is adaptive functioning that determines the level of supports required. Moreover, IQ measures are less valid in the lower end of the IQ range. This represents a change from DSM-IV, in which mental retardation severity levels were based on IQ scores.

**5—Intellectual Disability (Intellectual Developmental Disorder) / Specifiers (p. 33)**

6. Which of the following is *not* a diagnostic feature of intellectual disability (intellectual developmental disorder)?

   A. A full-scale IQ of less than 70.
   B. Inability to perform complex daily living tasks (e.g., money management, medical decision making) without support.

C. Gullibility, with naiveté in social situations and a tendency to be easily led by others.
D. Lack of age-appropriate communication skills for social and interpersonal functioning.
E. All of the above are diagnostic features of intellectual disability.

**Correct Answer: A. A full-scale IQ of less than 70.**

**Explanation:** The DSM-5 diagnosis does not require a full-scale IQ less than 70, because impairment in adaptive functioning is also required. In general, individuals with intellectual disability may have difficulty with social judgment. Lack of communication skills may also predispose them to disruptive and aggressive behaviors. Communication, conversation, and language are more concrete or immature than expected for any given age. Furthermore, gullibility is an important feature of intellectual developmental disorder. It is especially important in forensic situations and may affect judgment.

**6—Intellectual Disability (Intellectual Developmental Disorder) / Diagnostic Features (p. 37)**

7. Which of the following statements about adaptive functioning in the diagnosis of intellectual disability (intellectual developmental disorder) is *true*?

A. Adaptive functioning is based on an individual's IQ score.
B. "Deficits in adaptive functioning" refers to problems with motor coordination.
C. At least two domains of adaptive functioning must be impaired to meet Criterion B for the diagnosis of intellectual disability.
D. Adaptive functioning in intellectual disability tends to improve over time, although the threshold of cognitive capacities and associated developmental disorders can limit it.
E. Individuals diagnosed with intellectual disability in childhood will typically continue to meet criteria in adulthood even if their adaptive functioning improves.

**Correct Answer: D. Adaptive functioning tends to improve over time, although the threshold of cognitive capacities and associated developmental disorders can limit it.**

**Explanation:** In the DSM-5 diagnosis of intellectual disability (intellectual developmental disorder), unlike the DSM-IV diagnosis of mental retardation, the various levels of severity are defined on the basis of adaptive functioning rather than IQ scores alone, because it is adaptive functioning that determines the level of support required. Moreover, IQ measures are less valid in the lower end of the IQ range. Severity levels are meant to refer only to functioning at the time of the assessment, and they can change over time in a positive direction if the individual receives support and can develop compensatory strategies. Improvement in adaptive functioning can occur to a degree such that the individual no longer meets criteria for the diagnosis in adulthood.

> 7—Intellectual Disability (Intellectual Developmental Disorder) / Specifiers (pp. 33–36); Diagnostic Features (pp. 37–38); Development and Course (pp. 38–39)

8. Which of the following statements about development of and risk factors for intellectual disability (intellectual developmental disorder) is *true?*

    A. Intellectual developmental disorder should not be diagnosed in the presence of a known genetic syndrome, such as Lesch-Nyhan or Prader-Willi syndrome.
    B. Etiologies are confined to perinatal and postnatal factors and exclude prenatal events.
    C. In severe acquired forms of intellectual developmental disorder, onset may be abrupt following an illness (e.g., meningitis) or head trauma occurring during the developmental period.
    D. When intellectual disability results from a loss of previously acquired cognitive skills, as in severe traumatic brain injury (TBI), only the TBI diagnosis is assigned.
    E. Prenatal, perinatal, and postnatal etiologies of intellectual developmental disorder are demonstrable in approximately 33% of cases.

**Correct Answer: C. In severe acquired forms of intellectual developmental disorder, onset may be abrupt following an illness (e.g., meningitis) or head trauma occurring during the developmental period.**

**Explanation:** The presence of a known genetic syndrome is *not* exclusionary if the criteria for intellectual developmental disorder are met. Prenatal, perinatal, and postnatal etiologies are demonstrable in approximately 70% of cases. If the diagnosis results from TBI, both diagnoses are given.

> 8—Intellectual Disability (Intellectual Developmental Disorder) / Development and Course (pp. 38–39); Risk and Prognostic Factors (p. 39)

9. Which of the following statements about the developmental course of intellectual disability (intellectual developmental disorder) is *true?*

    A. Delayed motor, language, and social milestones are not identifiable until after the first 2 years of life.
    B. Intellectual disability caused by an illness (e.g., encephalitis) or by head trauma occurring during the developmental period would be diagnosed as a neurocognitive disorder, not as intellectual disability (intellectual developmental disorder).
    C. Intellectual disability is always nonprogressive.
    D. Major neurocognitive disorder may co-occur with intellectual developmental disorder.

E. Even if early and ongoing interventions throughout childhood and adulthood lead to improved adaptive and intellectual functioning, the diagnosis of intellectual disability would continue to apply.

**Correct Answer: D. Major neurocognitive disorder may co-occur with intellectual developmental disorder.**

**Explanation:** Intellectual disability is categorized as a neurodevelopmental disorder and is distinct from the neurocognitive disorders, which are characterized by a loss of cognitive functioning. Major neurocognitive disorder may co-occur with intellectual disability (e.g., an individual with Down syndrome who develops Alzheimer's disease, or an individual with intellectual disability who loses further cognitive capacity following a head injury). In such cases, the diagnoses of intellectual disability and neurocognitive disorder may both be given.

Delayed motor, language, and social milestones may be identifiable within the first 2 years of life among those with more severe intellectual disability. Head trauma with subsequent cognitive deficits would represent an acquired form of intellectual developmental disorders. Although intellectual disability is generally nonprogressive, in certain genetic disorders (e.g., Rett syndrome) there are periods of worsening, followed by stabilization, and in others (e.g., San Phillippo syndrome) progressive worsening of intellectual function. After early childhood, the disorder is generally lifelong, although severity levels may change over time. If early and ongoing interventions improve adaptive functioning and significant improvement of intellectual functioning occurs, the diagnosis of intellectual disability may no longer be appropriate.

> 9—Intellectual Disability (Intellectual Developmental Disorder) / Development and Course (pp. 38–39); Differential Diagnosis (pp. 39–40); Comorbidity (p. 40)

10. The DSM-5 diagnosis of intellectual developmental disorder includes severity specifiers—Mild, Moderate, Severe, and Profound—with which to indicate the level of supports required in various domains of adaptive functioning. Which of the following features would *not* be characteristic of an individual with a "Severe" level of impairment?

    A. The individual generally has little understanding of written language or of concepts involving numbers, quantity, time, and money.
    B. The individual's spoken language is quite limited in terms of vocabulary and grammar.
    C. The individual requires support for all activities of daily living, including meals, dressing, bathing, and toileting.
    D. In adulthood, the individual may be able to sustain competitive employment in a job that does not emphasize conceptual skills.
    E. The individual cannot make responsible decisions regarding the well-being of self or others.

**Correct Answer: D. In adulthood, the individual may be able to sustain competitive employment in a job that does not emphasize conceptual skills.**

**Explanation:** Competitive employment may be attainable by individuals with a "Mild" level of impairment but would not be characteristic of those with a "Severe" level of impairment. Intellectual disability (intellectual developmental disorder) is a disorder with onset during the developmental period that includes both intellectual and adaptive functioning deficits in conceptual, social, and practical domains (DSM-5 Table 1, pp. 34–36). The *conceptual (academic) domain* involves competence in memory, language, reading, writing, math reasoning, acquisition of practical knowledge, problem solving, and judgment in novel situations, among others. The *social domain* involves awareness of others' thoughts, feelings, and experiences; empathy; interpersonal communication skills; friendship abilities; and social judgment, among others. The *practical domain* involves learning and self-management across life settings, including personal care, job responsibilities, money management, recreation, self-management of behavior, and school and work task organization, among others.

> 10—Intellectual Disability (Intellectual Developmental Disorder) / diagnostic criteria (p. 33) / Table 1 [Severity levels for intellectual disability (intellectual developmental disorder)] (pp. 33–36); Diagnostic Features (p. 37)

11. A 10-year-old boy with a history of dyslexia, who is otherwise developmentally normal, is in a skateboarding accident in which he experiences severe traumatic brain injury. This results in significant global intellectual impairment (with a persistent reading deficit that is more pronounced than his other newly acquired but stable deficits, along with a full-scale IQ of 75). There is mild impairment in his adaptive functioning such that he requires support in some areas of functioning. He is also displaying anxious and depressive symptoms in response to his accident and hospitalization. What is the *least likely* diagnosis?

    A. Intellectual disability (intellectual developmental disorder).
    B. Traumatic brain injury.
    C. Specific learning disorder.
    D. Major neurocognitive disorder due to traumatic brain injury.
    E. Adjustment disorder.

**Correct Answer: D. Major neurocognitive disorder due to traumatic brain injury.**

**Explanation:** There are no exclusion criteria for a diagnosis of intellectual developmental disorder in DSM-5, which notes that both specific learning disorder and communication disorders can co-occur if the criteria are met. Although his full-scale IQ is 75, the statistical model associated with his intellect would allow for his actual IQ to be ±5 points. His adaptive functioning would be the key factor in his receiving the diagnosis of intellectual developmental disorder, with a mild level of severity due to needing to receive only some support in most of his areas of functioning. With his reading skills remaining disproportionately impaired in comparison with the rest of his cognitive profile, and because onset of these impairments was during the developmental period, he would continue to receive a diagnosis of specific learning disorder (dyslexia). His emotional symptoms in response to the accident would yield a potential diagnosis of an adjustment disorder. The boy's deficits are not severe enough to qualify for a diagnosis of major neurocognitive disorder.

**11—Intellectual Disability (Intellectual Developmental Disorder) / Differential Diagnosis (p. 40)**

12. In which of the following situations would a diagnosis of global developmental delay be *inappropriate?*

    A. The patient is a child who is too young to fully manifest specific symptoms or to complete requisite assessments.
    B. The patient, a 7-year-old boy, has a full-scale IQ of 65 and severe impairment in adaptive functioning.
    C. The patient's scores on psychometric tests suggest intellectual disability (intellectual developmental disorder), but there is insufficient information about the patient's adaptive functional skills.
    D. The patient's impaired adaptive functioning suggests intellectual developmental disorder, but there is insufficient information about the level of cognitive impairment measured by standardized instruments.
    E. The patient's cognitive and adaptive impairments suggest intellectual developmental disorder, but there is insufficient information about age at onset of the condition.

    **Correct Answer: B. The patient, a 7-year-old boy, has a full-scale IQ of 65 and severe impairment in adaptive functioning.**

    **Explanation:** Enough information is present to diagnose intellectual disability (intellectual developmental disorder) in this boy. The diagnosis of global developmental delay is used when there is insufficient information to make the diagnosis of intellectual developmental disorder.

    **12—Global Developmental Delay (p. 41)**

13. Which of the following statements about global developmental delay is *true?*

    A. The diagnosis is typically made in children younger than 5 years of age.
    B. The etiology can usually be determined.
    C. The prevalence is estimated to be between 0.5% and 2%.
    D. The condition is progressive.
    E. The condition does not generally occur with other neurodevelopmental disorders.

**Correct Answer: A. The diagnosis is typically made in children younger than 5 years of age.**

**Explanation:** The diagnosis of global developmental delay is reserved for individuals under the age of 5 years who fail to meet expected developmental milestones in several areas of intellectual functioning, when the clinical severity level cannot be reliably assessed during early childhood. The diagnosis is used for individuals who are unable to undergo systematic assessments of intellectual functioning, including children who are too young to participate in standardized testing.

**13—Global Developmental Delay (p. 41)**

14. A 3½-year-old girl with a history of lead exposure and a seizure disorder demonstrates substantial delays across multiple domains of functioning, including communication, learning, attention, and motor development, which limit her ability to interact with same-age peers and require substantial support in all activities of daily living at home. Unfortunately, her mother is an extremely poor historian, and the child has received no formal psychological or learning evaluation to date. She is about to be evaluated for readiness to attend preschool. What is the most appropriate diagnosis?

    A. Major neurocognitive disorder.
    B. Developmental coordination disorder.
    C. Autism spectrum disorder.
    D. Global developmental delay.
    E. Specific learning disorder.

**Correct Answer: D. Global developmental delay.**

**Explanation:** Although this girl's deficits may be suggestive of intellectual disability (intellectual developmental disorder), that diagnosis cannot be made in this case because information is lacking (e.g., about age at onset of her symptoms), and she is too young to participate in standardized testing. At this point, there is no information to suggest that this child has dementia (major neurocognitive disorder), an autism spectrum disorder (no evidence of symptoms in the core autism spectrum disorder categories), a specific disorder relating to coordination, or a specific area of learning weakness (which generally would not be able to be diagnosed until the elementary years).

**14—Global Developmental Delay (p. 41)**

15. A 5-year-old boy has difficulty making friends and problems with initiating and sustaining back-and-forth conversation; reading social cues; and sharing his feelings with others. He makes good eye contact, has normal speech intonation, displays facial gestures, and has a range of affect that generally seems appropriate to the situation. He demonstrates an interest in trains that seems

abnormal in intensity and focus, and he engages in little imaginative or symbolic play. Which of the following diagnostic requirements for autism spectrum disorder are *not* met in this case?

A. Deficits in social-emotional reciprocity.
B. Deficits in nonverbal communicative behaviors used for social interaction.
C. Deficits in developing and maintaining relationships.
D. Restricted, repetitive patterns of behavior, interests, or activities as manifested by symptoms in two of the specified four categories.
E. Symptoms with onset in early childhood that cause clinically significant impairment.

**Correct Answer: B. Deficits in nonverbal communicative behaviors used for social interaction.**

**Explanation:** DSM-5 Criterion A for autism spectrum disorder specifies that all three symptom clusters (summarized in options A, B, and C above) must be met. This boy's nonverbal communication is reported to be unimpaired (although this should be confirmed with a standard instrument such as the Autism Diagnostic Observation Schedule). Based on the current history, he could not be diagnosed with autism spectrum disorder in DSM-5. In order to meet Criterion B, at least two symptom clusters must be met. Although the boy has "highly restricted, fixated interests that are abnormal in intensity or focus," he would need to have at least one other symptom from categories in Criterion B (which includes stereotyped or repetitive motor movements, use of objects, or speech; insistence on sameness, inflexible adherence to routines, or ritualized patterns of verbal or nonverbal behavior; or hyper- or hyporeactivity to sensory input or unusual interest in sensory aspects of the environment).

**15—Autism Spectrum Disorder / diagnostic criteria (p. 50)**

16. Which of the following statements about the development and course of autism spectrum disorder (ASD) is *false?*

A. Symptoms of ASD are typically recognized during the second year of life (12–24 months of age).
B. Symptoms of ASD are usually not noticeable until 5–6 years of age or later.
C. First symptoms frequently involve delayed language development, often accompanied by lack of social interest or unusual social interactions.
D. ASD is not a degenerative disorder, and it is typical for learning and compensation to continue throughout life.
E. Because many normally developing young children have strong preferences and enjoy repetition, distinguishing restricted and repetitive behaviors that are diagnostic of ASD can be difficult in preschoolers.

**Correct Answer: B. Symptoms are not typically noticeable until 5–6 years of age or later.**

**Explanation:** Details about the age and pattern of onset are important and should be noted in the history. Symptoms of ASD are typically recognized during the second year of life (12–24 months of age) but may be seen earlier than 12 months if developmental delays are severe, or noted later than 24 months if symptoms are more subtle. The pattern of onset description might include information about early developmental delays or any losses of social or language skills. In cases where skills have been lost, parents or caregivers may give a history of a gradual or relatively rapid deterioration in social behaviors or language skills. Typically, this would occur between 12 and 24 months of age and is distinguished from the rare instances of developmental regression occurring after at least 2 years of normal development (previously described as childhood disintegrative disorder).

**16—Autism Spectrum Disorder / Development and Course (pp. 55–56)**

17. Which of the following was a criterion symptom for autistic disorder in DSM-IV that was eliminated from the diagnostic criteria for autism spectrum disorder in DSM-5?

    A. Stereotyped or restricted patterns of interest.
    B. Stereotyped and repetitive motor mannerisms.
    C. Inflexible adherence to routines.
    D. Persistent preoccupation with parts of objects.
    E. None of the above.

**Correct Answer: D. Persistent preoccupation with parts of objects.**

**Explanation:** In DSM-5, the older requirement regarding objects was restated as follows: "Highly restricted, fixated interests that are abnormal in intensity or focus (e.g., strong attachment to or preoccupation with unusual objects, excessively circumscribed or perseverative interests)" in Criterion B3. In Criterion B4, DSM-5 mentions "fascination with lights or spinning objects." There is no mention of preoccupation with "parts of objects" in DSM-5 (Criterion A3d in DSM-IV autistic disorder).

**17—Autism Spectrum Disorder / diagnostic criteria (p. 50)**

18. A 7-year-old girl presents with a history of normal language skills (vocabulary and grammar intact) but is unable to use language in a socially pragmatic manner to share ideas and feelings. She has never made good eye contact, and she has difficulty reading social cues. Consequently, she has had difficulty making friends, which is further complicated by her being somewhat obsessed with cartoon characters, which she repetitively scripts. She tends to excessively smell objects. Because she insists on wearing the same shirt and shorts every day, regardless of the season, getting dressed is a difficult activity. These symptoms date from early childhood and cause significant impairment in her functioning. What diagnosis best fits this child's presentation?

    A. Asperger's disorder.
    B. Autism spectrum disorder.
    C. Pervasive developmental disorder not otherwise specified (NOS).
    D. Social (pragmatic) communication disorder.
    E. Rett syndrome.

**Correct Answer: B. Autism spectrum disorder.**

**Explanation:** This child might have met criteria for Asperger's disorder or pervasive developmental disorder NOS in DSM-IV. Autism spectrum disorder in DSM-5 subsumed Asperger's disorder and pervasive developmental disorder NOS. Although the girl has intact formal language skills, it is the use of language for social communication that is particularly affected in autism spectrum disorder. A specific language delay is not required. She meets all three components of Criterion A (deficits in social-emotional reciprocity, deficits in nonverbal communicative behaviors used for social interaction, and deficits in developing, maintaining, and understanding relationships) and two components of Criterion B (highly restricted, fixated interests that are abnormal in intensity or focus; and hyper- or hyporeactivity to sensory input or unusual interest in sensory aspects of the environment).

**18—Autism Spectrum Disorder / Diagnostic Features (p. 53)**

19. A 15-year-old boy has a long history of nonverbal communication deficits. As an infant he was unable to follow someone else directing his attention by pointing. As a toddler he was not interested in sharing events, feelings, or games with his parents. From school age into adolescence, his speech was odd in tonality and phrasing, and his body language was awkward. What do these symptoms represent?

    A. Stereotypies.
    B. Restricted range of interests.
    C. Developmental regression.
    D. Prodromal schizophreniform symptoms.
    E. Deficits in nonverbal communicative behaviors.

**Correct Answer: E. Deficits in nonverbal communicative behaviors.**

**Explanation:** These symptoms are examples of deficits in nonverbal communicative behavior, as described in Criterion A2 for autism spectrum disorder criteria in DSM-5.

**19—Autism Spectrum Disorder / Diagnostic Features (p. 53)**

20. A 10-year-old boy demonstrates hand-flapping and finger flicking, and he repetitively flips coins and lines up his trucks. He tends to "echo" the last several words of a question posed to him before answering, mixes up his pronouns (re-

fers to himself in the second person), tends to repeat phrases in a perseverative fashion, and is quite fixated on routines related to dress, eating, travel, and play. He spends hours in his garage playing with his father's tools. What do these behaviors represent?

A. Restricted, repetitive patterns of behaviors, interests, or activities characteristic of autism spectrum disorder.
B. Symptoms of obsessive-compulsive disorder.
C. Prototypical manifestations of obsessive-compulsive personality.
D. Symptoms of pediatric acute-onset neuropsychiatric syndrome (PANS).
E. Complex tics.

**Correct Answer: A. Restricted, repetitive patterns of behaviors, interests, or activities characteristic of autism spectrum disorder.**

**Explanation:** In DSM-5, the symptoms in the category of "restrictive, repetitive patterns of behaviors, interests, or activities" (Criterion B) associated with autism spectrum disorder demonstrated by this patient include stereotyped or repetitive motor movements, use of objects, or speech; insistence on sameness, inflexible adherence to routines, or ritualized patterns of verbal or nonverbal behavior; and highly restricted, fixated interests that are abnormal in intensity or focus. He needs to have only two out of the four symptoms in this category (along with meeting Criterion A) to qualify for the autism spectrum disorder diagnosis. The fourth symptom in Criterion B (which this patient does not display) is hyper- or hyporeactivity to sensory input or unusual interest in sensory aspects of the environment.

**20—Autism Spectrum Disorder / Diagnostic Features (p. 53)**

21. A 25-year-old man presents with long-standing nonverbal communication deficits, inability to have a back-and-forth conversation or share interests in an appropriate fashion, and a complete lack of interest in having relationships with others. His speech reflects awkward phrasing and intonation and is mechanical in nature. He has a history of sequential fixations and obsessions with various games and objects throughout childhood; however, this is not currently a major issue for him. This patient meets criteria for autism spectrum disorder; true or false?

A. True.
B. False.

**Correct Answer: A. True.**

**Explanation:** This young man presents with all three symptoms in Criterion A; his symptoms satisfy Criterion C, which requires childhood onset; and he meets Criterion D, which requires clinically significant impairment in functioning. Although he has only one symptom in Criterion B (stereotyped or repetitive speech) and the diagnosis requires two, the fact that he has a history of fixations and obsessions satisfies the criteria, such that he does qualify for a diagnosis of autism spectrum disorder.

**21—Autism Spectrum Disorder / diagnostic criteria (p. 50)**

22. A 9-year-old girl presents with a history of intellectual impairment, a structural language impairment, nonverbal communication deficits, disinterest in peers, and inability to use language in a social manner. She has extreme food and tactile sensitivities. She is obsessed with one particular computer game that she plays for hours each day, and she scripts and imitates the characters in this game. She is clumsy, has an odd gait, and walks on her tiptoes. In the past year she has developed a seizure disorder and has begun to bang her wrists against the wall repetitively, causing bruising. On the other hand, she plays several musical instruments in an extremely precocious manner. Which feature of this child's clinical presentation fulfills a criterion symptom for DSM-5 autism spectrum disorder?

    A. Motor abnormalities.
    B. Seizures.
    C. Structural language impairment.
    D. Intellectual impairment.
    E. Nonverbal communicative deficits.

    **Correct Answer: E. Nonverbal communicative deficits.**

    **Explanation:** Criterion A of autism spectrum disorder lists nonverbal communicative deficits as one of the symptoms. The rest of the options represent associated features supporting diagnosis, which according to the DSM-5 text notes that "the gap between intellectual and adaptive functional skills is often large."

    **22—Autism Spectrum Disorder / diagnostic criteria (p. 50); Associated Features Supporting Diagnosis (p. 55)**

23. An 11-year-old girl with autism spectrum disorder displays no spoken language and is minimally responsive to overtures from others. She can be somewhat inflexible, which interferes with her ability to travel, do schoolwork, and be managed in the home; she has some difficulty transitioning; and she has trouble organizing and planning activities. These problems can usually be managed with incentives and reinforcers. What severity levels should be specified in the DSM-5 diagnosis?

    A. Level 3 (requiring very substantial support) for social communication, and level 1 (requiring support) for restricted, repetitive behaviors.
    B. Level 1 (requiring support) for social communication, and level 3 (requiring very substantial support) for restricted, repetitive behaviors.
    C. Level 1 (requiring support) for social communication, and level 2 (requiring substantial support) for restricted, repetitive behaviors.

D. Level 3 (requiring very substantial support) for social communication, and level 1 (requiring support) for restricted, repetitive behaviors.

E. Level 2 (requiring substantial support) for social communication, and level 1 (requiring support) for restricted, repetitive behaviors.

**Correct Answer: A. Level 3 (requiring very substantial support) for social communication, and level 1 (requiring support) for restricted, repetitive behaviors.**

**Explanation:** In DSM-5, severity is noted separately for social communication impairments and for the restricted, repetitive patterns of behavior. In this case, the social communication deficits are quite severe, warranting a classification of level 3, but the restricted, repetitive behaviors are milder, reflecting the lowest classification of level 1. Level 2 is an intermediate category reflecting the need for "substantial support."

**23—Autism Spectrum Disorder / Specifiers (p. 51)**

24. Which of the following is *not* a specifier included in the diagnostic criteria for autism spectrum disorder?

A. With or without accompanying intellectual impairment.
B. With or without associated dementia.
C. With or without accompanying language impairment.
D. Associated with a known medical or genetic condition or environmental factor.
E. Associated with another neurodevelopmental, mental, or behavioral disorder.

**Correct Answer: B. With or without associated dementia.**

**Explanation:** The specifier "with or without associated dementia" is not included in the diagnostic criteria for autism spectrum disorder.

**24—Autism Spectrum Disorder / diagnostic criteria (p. 51)**

25. Which of the following is *not* characteristic of the developmental course of children diagnosed with autism spectrum disorder?

A. Behavioral features manifest before 3 years of age.
B. The full symptom pattern does not appear until age 2–3 years.
C. Developmental plateaus or regression in social-communicative behavior is frequently reported by parents.
D. Regression across multiple domains occurs after age 2–3 years.
E. First symptoms often include delayed language development, lack of social interest or unusual social behavior, odd play, and unusual communication patterns.

**Correct Answer: D. Regression across multiple domains occurs after age 2–3 years.**

**Explanation:** Regression across multiple domains after age 2–3 years may occur, but it is not typical of the developmental course in autism spectrum disorder. As noted in DSM-5, some children with autism spectrum disorder experience developmental plateaus or regression, with a gradual or relatively rapid deterioration in social behaviors or use of language, often during the first 2 years of life. Such losses are rare in other disorders and may be a useful "red flag" for autism spectrum disorder. Much more unusual and warranting more extensive medical investigation are losses of skills beyond social communication (e.g., loss of self-care, toileting, motor skills) or those occurring after the second birthday.

**25—Autism Spectrum Disorder / Development and Course (pp. 55–56)**

26. A 5-year-old girl has some mild food aversions. She enjoys having the same book read to her at night but does not become terribly upset if her mother asks her to choose a different book. She occasionally spins around excitedly when her favorite show is on. She generally likes her toys neatly arranged in bins but is only mildly upset when her sister leaves them on the floor. These behaviors should be considered suspicious for an autism spectrum disorder; true or false?

A. True.
B. False.

**Correct Answer: B. False.**

**Explanation:** The girl described in the question meets none of the criteria for autism spectrum disorder. Because many typically developing young children have strong preferences and enjoy repetition (e.g., eating the same foods, watching the same video multiple times), distinguishing restricted and repetitive behaviors that are diagnostic of autism spectrum disorder can be difficult in preschoolers. The clinical distinction is based on the type, frequency, and intensity of the behavior (e.g., a child who daily lines up objects for hours and is very distressed if any item is moved).

**26—Autism Spectrum Disorder / Development and Course (p. 56)**

27. Which of the following is *not* representative of the typical developmental course for autism spectrum disorder?

A. Lack of degenerative course.
B. Behavioral deterioration during adolescence.
C. Continued learning and compensation throughout life.

D. Marked presence of symptoms in early childhood and early school years, with developmental gains in later childhood in areas such as social interaction.

E. Good psychosocial functioning in adulthood, as indexed by independent living and gainful employment.

**Correct Answer: B. Behavioral deterioration during adolescence.**

**Explanation:** Most adolescents with autism spectrum disorder improve behaviorally; only a minority further deteriorates.

**27—Autism Spectrum Disorder / Development and Course (pp. 55–56)**

28. A 21-year-old man, not previously diagnosed with a developmental disorder, presents for evaluation after taking a leave from college for psychological reasons. He makes little eye contact, does not appear to pick up on social cues, has become disinterested in friends, spends hours each day on the computer surfing the Internet and playing games, and has become so sensitive to smells that he keeps multiple air fresheners in all locations of the home. He reports that he has had long-standing friendships dating from childhood and high school (corroborated by his parents). He reports making many friends in his fraternity at college. His parents report good social and communication skills in childhood, although he was quite shy and was somewhat inflexible and ritualistic at home. What is the *least likely* diagnosis?

A. Depression.
B. Schizophreniform disorder or schizophrenia.
C. Autism spectrum disorder.
D. Obsessive-compulsive disorder.
E. Social anxiety disorder (social phobia).

**Correct Answer: C. Autism spectrum disorder.**

**Explanation:** The history of good social and communication skills in childhood and long-standing friendships is not consistent with autism spectrum disorder. With respect to schizophrenia specifically, DSM-5 text notes that "schizophrenia with childhood onset usually develops after a period of normal, or near normal, development. A prodromal state has been described in which social impairment and atypical interests and beliefs occur, which could be confused with the social deficits seen in autism spectrum disorder. Hallucinations and delusions, which are defining features of schizophrenia, are not features of autism spectrum disorder."

**28—Autism Spectrum Disorder / Differential Diagnosis (p. 58)**

29. Which of the following characteristics is generally *not* associated with autism spectrum disorder?

   A. Anxiety, depression, and isolation as an adult.
   B. Catatonia.
   C. Poor psychosocial functioning.
   D. Insistence on routines and aversion to change.
   E. Successful adaptation in regular school settings.

**Correct Answer: E. Successful adaptation in regular school settings.**

**Explanation:** In young children with autism spectrum disorder, lack of social and communication abilities may hamper learning, especially learning through social interaction or in settings with peers. In the home, insistence on routines and aversion to change, as well as sensory sensitivities, may interfere with eating and sleeping and make routine care (e.g., haircuts, dental work) extremely difficult. Adaptive skills are typically below measured IQ. Extreme difficulties in planning, organization, and coping with change negatively impact academic achievement, even for students with above-average intelligence. During adulthood, these individuals may have difficulties establishing independence because of continued rigidity and difficulty with novelty.

**29—Autism Spectrum Disorder / Functional Consequences of Autism Spectrum Disorder (p. 57)**

30. Which of the following disorders is generally *not* comorbid with autism spectrum disorder (ASD)?

   A. Attention-deficit/hyperactivity disorder (ADHD).
   B. Rett syndrome.
   C. Selective mutism.
   D. Intellectual disability (intellectual developmental disorder).
   E. Stereotypic movement disorder.

**Correct Answer: C. Selective mutism.**

**Explanation:** Children with selective mutism have appropriate communication skills in certain contexts and do not demonstrate severe impairments in social interaction and restricted patterns of behavior; in selective mutism, there are typically no abnormalities in early development, and no restricted and repetitive behavior or interests. ADHD can be comorbid with ASD in DSM-5 (unlike in DSM-IV); such comorbidity would be coded with the specifier "associated with another neurodevelopmental, mental, or behavioral disorder." ASD and Rett syndrome can be comorbid, with Rett syndrome similarly coded as the associated "known medical or genetic condition or environmental factor," as long as the child also meets criteria for autism spectrum disorder. ASD can be comorbid with intellectual developmental disorder when all criteria for both disorders are met, and "social communication and interaction are significantly impaired relative to the developmental level of the individual's nonverbal skills," that is, there is a discrepancy between social-communicative skills and nonverbal skills. ASD can be comorbid with stereotypic movement disorder if the repetitive movements cannot be accounted for as part of the autism spectrum disorder (e.g., hand flapping). In general, when criteria for another disorder are met along with meeting the criteria for ASD, both disorders are diagnosed. Comorbidity with additional diagnoses in ASD is common (about 70% of individuals with autism spectrum disorder have one comorbid mental disorder, and 40% have two or more comorbid mental disorders).

**30—Autism Spectrum Disorder / Comorbidity (pp. 58–59)**

31. Which of the following is *not* a criterion for the DSM-5 diagnosis of attention-deficit/hyperactivity disorder (ADHD)?

    A. Onset of several inattentive or hyperactive-impulsive symptoms prior to age 12 years.
    B. Manifestation of several inattentive or hyperactive-impulsive symptoms in two or more settings (e.g., at home, school, or work; with friends or relatives; in other activities).
    C. Persistence of symptoms for at least 12 months.
    D. Clear evidence that symptoms interfere with, or reduce the quality of, social, academic, or occupational functioning.
    E. Inability to explain symptoms as a manifestation of another mental disorder (e.g., mood disorder, anxiety disorder, dissociative disorder, personality disorder, substance intoxication or withdrawal).

**Correct Answer: C. Persistence of symptoms for at least 12 months.**

**Explanation:** The essential feature of ADHD is a pervasive pattern of *inattention* and/or *hyperactivity-impulsivity* that interferes with functioning or development, with persistence of symptoms for at least 6 months to a degree that is inconsistent with developmental level and that negatively impacts directly on social and academic/occupational activities. ADHD begins in childhood. The requirement that several symptoms be present before age 12 years conveys the importance of a substantial clinical presentation during childhood. Manifestations of the disorder must be present in more than one setting (e.g., home and school, work). Confirmation of substantial symptoms across settings typically cannot be done accurately without consulting informants who have seen the individual in those settings.

**31—Attention-Deficit/Hyperactivity Disorder / diagnostic criteria (p. 59); Diagnostic Features (p. 61)**

32. The parents of a 15-year-old female tenth grader believe that she should be doing better in high school, given how bright she seems and the fact that she received mostly A's through eighth grade. Her papers are handed in late, and she makes careless mistakes on examinations. They have her tested, and the WAIS-IV results are as follows: Verbal IQ, 125; Perceptual Reasoning Index, 122; Full-Scale IQ, 123; Working Memory Index, 55th percentile; Processing Speed Index, 50th percentile. Weaknesses in executive function are noted. During a psychiatric evaluation, she reports a long history of failing to give close attention to details, difficulty sustaining attention while in class or doing homework, failing to finish chores and tasks, and significant difficulties with time management, planning, and organization. She is forgetful, often loses things, and is easily distracted. She has no history of restlessness or impulsivity, and she is well liked by her peers. What is the most likely diagnosis?

    A. Adjustment disorder with anxiety.
    B. Specific learning disorder.
    C. Attention-deficit/hyperactivity disorder, predominantly inattentive.
    D. Developmental coordination disorder.
    E. Major depressive disorder.

    **Correct Answer: C. Attention-deficit/hyperactivity disorder, predominantly inattentive.**

    **Explanation:** The patient has six symptoms in the inattention cluster of attention-deficit/hyperactivity disorder (ADHD) and meets criteria for this disorder. She has common associated features of ADHD, including weaknesses in working memory and processing speed, and problems handing in her work (especially writing) on time. There is no evidence from the testing or history that her writing difficulty is secondary to a primary disorder involving writing or that she has any other specific learning disorder.

    **32—Attention-Deficit/Hyperactivity Disorder / Differential Diagnosis (p. 63)**

33. A 7-year-old boy is having behavioral and social difficulties in his second-grade class. Although he seems to be able to attend and is doing "well" from an academic standpoint (though seemingly not what he is capable of), he is constantly interrupting, fidgeting, talking excessively, and getting out of his seat. He has friends, but he sometimes annoys his peers because of his difficulty sharing and taking turns and the fact that he is constantly talking over them. Although he seeks out play dates, his friends tire of him because he wants to play sports nonstop. At home, he can barely stay in his seat for a meal and is unable to play quietly. Although he shows remorse when the consequences of his behavior are pointed out to him, he can become angry in response and seems nevertheless unable to inhibit himself. What is the most likely diagnosis?

    A. Bipolar disorder.
    B. Autism spectrum disorder.

C. Generalized anxiety disorder.

D. Attention-deficit/hyperactivity disorder, predominantly hyperactive/impulsive.

E. Specific learning disorder.

**Correct Answer: D. Attention-deficit/hyperactivity disorder, predominantly hyperactive/impulsive.**

**Explanation:** This boy has all the cardinal features in the hyperactivity/impulsivity cluster of attention-deficit/hyperactivity disorder (ADHD). Although he is not currently displaying inattention or impairment in his academic functioning, it is quite likely that this will become more of an issue as schoolwork becomes more complex and tedious, and academic demands increase. His behaviors are somewhat alienating to peers, as is common in ADHD. There is no evidence that he has comorbid autism spectrum disorder, especially because he seeks out friendships. He meets Criterion C in that "several inattentive or hyperactive-impulsive symptoms are present in two or more settings (e.g., at home, school, or work; with friends or relatives; in other activities)" and Criterion D in that "there is clear evidence that the symptoms interfere with, or reduce the quality of, social, academic, or occupational functioning."

**33—Attention-Deficit/Hyperactivity Disorder / Differential Diagnosis (p. 63)**

34. A 37-year-old Wall Street trader schedules a visit after his 8-year-old son is diagnosed with attention-deficit/hyperactivity disorder (ADHD), combined inattentive and hyperactive. Although he does not currently note motor restlessness like his son, he recalls being that way when he was a boy, along with being quite inattentive, being impulsive, talking excessively, interrupting, and having problems waiting his turn. He was an underachiever in high school and college, when he inconsistently did his work and had difficulty following rules. Nevertheless, he never failed any classes, and he was never evaluated by a psychologist or psychiatrist. He works about 60–80 hours a week and often gets insufficient sleep. He tends to make impulsive business decisions, can be impatient and short-tempered, and notes that his mind tends to wander both in one-on-one interactions with associates and his wife and during business meetings, for which he is often late; he is forgetful and disorganized. Nevertheless, he tends to perform fairly well and is quite successful, although he can occasionally feel overwhelmed and demoralized. What is the most likely diagnosis?

A. Major depressive disorder.

B. Generalized anxiety disorder.

C. Specific learning disorder.

D. ADHD, in partial remission.

E. Oppositional defiant disorder.

**Correct Answer: D. ADHD, in partial remission.**

**Explanation:** This is a not uncommon story of a parent who presents to treatment after a son or daughter is diagnosed with ADHD, and the parent recognizes similarities from his or her own childhood. This man does present with a possible history of ADHD during childhood, along with a possible *prior* history of oppositional defiant disorder. Currently, there is no evidence that he has difficulty with rules, and the fact that he is no longer restless is common for the developmental course of ADHD. Currently, his ADHD symptoms include three symptoms in the inattention cluster (difficulty sustaining attention, difficulty organizing tasks and activities, forgetfulness), and only one clear symptom of impulsivity (impatience); since he has retained only some of the symptoms, a diagnosis of ADHD, *in partial remission,* is appropriate and provided for in DSM-5. It is unclear to what degree his work schedule and insufficient sleep are also contributing to his distress.

**34—Attention-Deficit/Hyperactivity Disorder / Differential Diagnosis (p. 63)**

35. A 5-year-old hyperactive, impulsive, and inattentive boy presents with hypertelorism, highly arched palate, and low-set ears. He is uncoordinated and clumsy, he has no sense of time, and his toys and clothes are constantly strewn all over the house. He has recently developed what appears to be a motor tic involving blinking. He enjoys playing with peers, who tend to like him, although he seems to willfully defy all requests from his parents and kindergarten teacher, which does not seem to be due simply to inattention. He is delayed in beginning to learn how to read. What is the *least likely* diagnosis?

    A. Autism spectrum disorder.
    B. Developmental coordination disorder.
    C. Oppositional defiant disorder (ODD).
    D. Specific learning disorder.
    E. Attention-deficit/hyperactivity disorder (ADHD).

**Correct Answer: A. Autism spectrum disorder.**

**Explanation:** There is no evidence that this boy has a disorder of relatedness, especially since he enjoys playing with peers, who like him. He has signs and symptoms of ADHD, along with some soft neurological signs and minor physical anomalies that can be associated with ADHD (although genetic and neurological evaluations seem warranted). He may have an associated specific learning disorder in reading (which should also be evaluated by having him tested by a psychologist) and a comorbid diagnosis of ODD, since his oppositional behavior is not simply due to inattention.

**35—Attention-Deficit/Hyperactivity Disorder / Differential Diagnosis (p. 63)**

36. What is the prevalence of attention-deficit/hyperactivity disorder (ADHD) in children?

    A. 8%.
    B. 10%.
    C. 2%.
    D. 0.5%.
    E. 5%.

**Correct Answer: E. 5%.**

**Explanation:** Population surveys suggest that ADHD occurs in most cultures in about 5% of children. Differences in ADHD prevalence rates across regions appear attributable mainly to different diagnostic and methodological practices. However, there also may be cultural variation in attitudes toward or interpretations of children's behaviors. Clinical identification rates in the United States for African American and Latino populations tend to be lower than for Caucasian populations. Informant symptom ratings may be influenced by the cultural group of the child and the informant, suggesting that culturally appropriate practices are relevant in assessing ADHD.

**36—Attention-Deficit/Hyperactivity Disorder / Prevalence (p. 61); Culture-Related Diagnostic Issues (p. 62)**

37. What is the prevalence of attention-deficit/hyperactivity disorder (ADHD) in adults?

    A. 8%.
    B. 10%.
    C. 2.5%.
    D. 0.5%.
    E. 5%.

**Correct Answer: C. 2.5%.**

**Explanation:** Population surveys suggest that ADHD occurs in most cultures in about 2.5% of adults and about 5% of children.

**37—Attention-Deficit/Hyperactivity Disorder / Prevalence (p. 61)**

38. What is the gender ratio of attention-deficit/hyperactivity disorder (ADHD) in children?

    A. Male:female ratio of 2:1.
    B. Male:female ratio of 1:1.
    C. Male:female ratio of 3:2.
    D. Male:female ratio of 5:1.
    E. Male:female ratio of 1:2.

**Correct Answer: A. Male:female ratio of 2:1.**

**Explanation:** ADHD is more prevalent in males than in females in the general population, with a gender ratio of approximately 2:1 in children and 1.6:1 in adults. Females are more likely than males to present primarily with inattentive features.

**38—Attention-Deficit/Hyperactivity Disorder / Gender-Related Diagnostic Issues (p. 63)**

39. Which of the following is a biological finding in individuals with attention-deficit/hyperactivity disorder (ADHD)?

    A. Decreased slow-wave activity on electroencephalograms.
    B. Reduced total brain volume on magnetic resonance imaging.
    C. Early posterior to anterior cortical maturation.
    D. Reduced thalamic volume.
    E. Both B and C.

    **Correct Answer: B. Reduced total brain volume on magnetic resonance imaging.**

    **Explanation:** No biological marker is diagnostic for ADHD. As a group, compared with peers, children with ADHD display reduced total brain volume on magnetic resonance imaging, *increased* slow-wave electroencephalograms, and possibly *a delay in* posterior to anterior cortical maturation.

    **39—Attention-Deficit/Hyperactivity Disorder / Associated Features Supporting Diagnosis (p. 61)**

40. Which of the following is *not* associated with attention-deficit/hyperactivity disorder (ADHD)?

    A. Reduced school performance.
    B. Poorer occupational performance and attendance.
    C. Higher probability of unemployment.
    D. Elevated interpersonal conflict.
    E. Reduced risk of substance use disorders.

    **Correct Answer: E. Reduced risk of substance use disorders.**

    **Explanation:** Children with ADHD are significantly more likely than their peers without ADHD to develop conduct disorder in adolescence and antisocial personality disorder in adulthood, consequently increasing the likelihood for substance use disorders and incarceration. The risk of subsequent substance use disorders is elevated, especially when conduct disorder or antisocial personality disorder develops.

    **40—Attention-Deficit/Hyperactivity Disorder / Functional Consequences of Attention-Deficit/Hyperactivity Disorder (p. 63)**

41. Which of the following is *not* associated with attention-deficit/hyperactivity disorder (ADHD)?

    A. Social rejection.
    B. Increased risk of developing conduct disorder in childhood and antisocial personality disorder in adulthood.
    C. Increased risk of Alzheimer's disease.
    D. Increased frequency of traffic accidents and violations.
    E. Increased risk of accidental injury.

    **Correct Answer: C. Increased risk of Alzheimer's disease.**

    **Explanation:** The risk of Alzheimer's disease is not elevated in individuals with ADHD. Peer relationships in individuals with ADHD are often disrupted by peer rejection, neglect, or teasing. Children with ADHD are significantly more likely than their peers without ADHD to develop conduct disorder in adolescence and antisocial personality disorder in adulthood, consequently increasing the likelihood for substance use disorders and incarceration. Individuals with ADHD are more likely than peers to be injured. Traffic accidents and violations are more frequent in drivers with ADHD.

    **41—Attention-Deficit/Hyperactivity Disorder / Functional Consequences of Attention-Deficit/Hyperactivity Disorder (p. 63)**

42. A 15-year-old boy has developed concentration problems in school that have been associated with a significant decline in grades. When interviewed, he explains that his mind is occupied with worrying about his mother, who has a serious autoimmune disease. As his grades falter, he becomes increasingly demoralized and sad, and he notices that his energy level drops, further compromising his ability to pay attention in school. At the same time, he complains of feeling restless and unable to sleep. What is the most likely diagnosis?

    A. Bipolar disorder.
    B. Specific learning disorder.
    C. Attention-deficit/hyperactivity disorder (ADHD).
    D. Adjustment disorder with mixed anxiety and depressed mood.
    E. Separation anxiety disorder.

    **Correct Answer: D. Adjustment disorder with mixed anxiety and depressed mood.**

    **Explanation:** The inattention seen in this boy relates to anxiety and depressive symptoms that are in reaction to his mother's illness and his subsequent decline in grades. Inattention related to ADHD is not associated with worry and rumination, as would be the case in anxiety disorders.

    **42—Attention-Deficit/Hyperactivity Disorder / Differential Diagnosis (p. 64)**

43. A 5-year-old boy is consistently moody, irritable, and intolerant of frustration. In addition, he is pervasively and chronically restless, impulsive, and inattentive. Which diagnosis best fits his clinical picture?

    A. Attention-deficit/hyperactivity disorder (ADHD).
    B. ADHD and disruptive mood dysregulation disorder (DMDD).
    C. Bipolar disorder.
    D. Oppositional defiant disorder (ODD).
    E. Major depressive disorder (MDD).

    **Correct Answer: B. ADHD and DMDD.**

    **Explanation:** The boy's mood symptoms cannot be accounted for by ADHD alone, and they are characteristic of DMDD; ADHD is not associated with this level of affective symptoms on its own. A diagnosis of bipolar disorder in this age group should be made extremely cautiously, given that less than 1% of preadolescent referrals have this diagnosis, especially when the cycles of "mania" last less than a day. Young people with bipolar disorder may have increased activity, but this is episodic, varying with mood, and goal directed. Therefore, this child's irritability and hyperactivity do not qualify for bipolar disorder.

    **43—Attention-Deficit/Hyperactivity Disorder / Differential Diagnosis (p. 64)**

44. Which of the following statements about comorbidity in attention-deficit/hyperactivity disorder (ADHD) is *true*?

    A. Oppositional defiant disorder co-occurs with ADHD in about half of children with the combined presentation and about a quarter of those with the predominantly inattentive presentation.
    B. Most children with disruptive mood dysregulation disorder do not also meet criteria for ADHD.
    C. Fifteen percent of adults with ADHD have some type of anxiety disorder.
    D. Intermittent explosive disorder occurs in about 5% of adults with ADHD.
    E. Specific learning disorder very seldom co-occurs with ADHD.

    **Correct Answer: A. Oppositional defiant disorder co-occurs with ADHD in about half of children with the combined presentation and about a quarter of those with the predominantly inattentive presentation.**

    **Explanation:** In clinical settings, comorbid disorders are frequent in individuals whose symptoms meet criteria for ADHD. In the general population, oppositional defiant disorder co-occurs with ADHD in approximately half of children with the combined presentation and about a quarter with the predominantly inattentive presentation. Most children and adolescents with disruptive mood dysregulation disorder have symptoms that also meet criteria for ADHD; a lesser percentage of children with ADHD have symptoms that meet criteria for disruptive mood dysregulation disorder. Specific learning disorder commonly co-occurs with ADHD. Anxiety disorders and major depressive disorder occur in a minority of individuals with ADHD but more often than in the general population. Intermittent explosive disorder occurs in a minority of adults with ADHD, but at rates above population levels. In adults, antisocial and other personality disorders may co-occur with ADHD. Other disorders that may co-occur with ADHD include obsessive-compulsive disorder, tic disorders, and autism spectrum disorder.

**44—Attention-Deficit/Hyperactivity Disorder / Comorbidity (p. 65)**

45. Specific learning disorder is defined by persistent difficulties in learning academic skills, with onset during the developmental period. Which of the following statements about this disorder is *true?*

    A. It is part of a more general learning impairment as manifested in intellectual disability (intellectual developmental disorder).
    B. It can usually be attributed to a sensory, physical, or neurological disorder.
    C. It involves pervasive and wide-ranging deficits across multiple domains of information processing.
    D. It can be caused by external factors such as economic disadvantage or lack of education.
    E. It replaces the DSM-IV diagnoses of reading disorder, mathematics disorder, disorder of written expression, and learning disorder not otherwise specified.

**Correct Answer: E. It replaces the DSM-IV diagnoses of reading disorder, mathematics disorder, disorder of written expression, and learning disorder not otherwise specified.**

**Explanation:** The DSM-5 diagnosis of specific learning disorder combines the DSM-IV diagnoses of reading disorder, mathematics disorder, disorder of written expression, and learning disorder not otherwise specified. The difficulties seen in specific learning disorder are considered "specific" for four reasons. First, they are not attributable to intellectual disabilities (intellectual disability [intellectual developmental disorder]); global developmental delay; hearing or vision disorders, or neurological or motor disorders) (Criterion D). Second, the learning difficulty cannot be attributed to more general external factors, such as economic or environmental disadvantage, chronic absenteeism, or lack of education as typically provided in the individual's community context. Third, the learning difficulty cannot be attributed to a neurological (e.g., pediatric stroke) or motor disorder or to vision or hearing disorders, which are often associated with problems learning academic skills but are distinguishable by presence of neurological signs. Finally, the learning difficulty may be restricted to one academic skill or domain (e.g., reading single words, retrieving or calculating number facts).

**45—Specific Learning Disorder / diagnostic criteria (p. 66); Diagnostic Features (pp. 69–70)**

46. In distinction to DSM-IV, DSM-5 classifies all learning disorders under the diagnosis of specific learning disorder, along with the requirement to "specify all academic domains and subskills that are impaired" at the time of assessment. Which of the following statements about specific learning disorder is *false?*

    A. There are persistent difficulties in the acquisition of reading, writing, arithmetic, or mathematical reasoning skills during the formal years of schooling.
    B. Current skills in one or more of these academic areas are well below the average range for the individual's age, gender, cultural group, and level of education.
    C. There usually is a discrepancy of more than 2 standard deviations (SD) between achievement and IQ.
    D. The learning difficulties significantly interfere with academic achievement, occupational performance, or activities of daily living that require these academic skills.
    E. The learning difficulties cannot be acquired later in life.

**Correct Answer: C. There usually is a discrepancy of more than 2 standard deviations (SD) between achievement and IQ.**

**Explanation:** DSM-IV stipulated that the individual's achievement on standardized tests be "substantially below" that expected for age, schooling, and level of intelligence. DSM-5 text further clarifies that academic skills are distributed along a continuum, so there is no natural cutpoint that can be used to differentiate individuals with and without specific learning disorder. Thus, any threshold used to specify what constitutes significantly low academic achievement (e.g., academic skills well below age expectation) is to a large extent arbitrary. Low achievement scores on one or more standardized tests or subtests within an academic domain (i.e., at least 1.5 SD below the population mean for age, which translates to a standard score ≤78, which is below the 7th percentile) are needed for the greatest diagnostic certainty. However, precise scores will vary according to the particular standardized tests that are used. Based on clinical judgment, a more lenient threshold may be used (e.g., 1.0–2.5 SD below the population mean for age), when learning difficulties are supported by converging evidence from clinical assessment, academic history, school reports, or test scores. Moreover, since standardized tests are not available in all languages, the diagnosis may then be based in part on clinical judgment of scores on available test measures.

46—Specific Learning Disorder / Diagnostic Features (p. 68)

47. Which of the following statements about the diagnosis of specific learning disorder is *false?*

    A. Specific learning disorder is distinct from learning problems associated with a neurodegenerative cognitive disorder.
    B. If intellectual disability (intellectual developmental disorder) is present, the learning difficulties must be in excess of those expected.
    C. An uneven profile of abilities is typical in specific learning disorder.
    D. Attentional difficulties and motor clumsiness that are subthreshold for attention-deficit/hyperactivity disorder or developmental coordination disorder are frequently associated with specific learning disorder.
    E. There are four formal subtypes of specific learning disorder.

**Correct Answer: E. There are four formal subtypes of specific learning disorder.**

**Explanation:** In DSM-5, there are no formal subtypes of specific learning disorder. Learning deficits in the areas of reading, written expression, and mathematics are coded as separate specifiers.

**47—Specific Learning Disorder / Differential Diagnosis (p. 73)**

48. Which of the following statements about prevalence rates for specific learning disorder is *false?*

    A. Prevalence rates range from 5% to 15% among school-age children across languages and cultures.
    B. Prevalence in adults is approximately 4%.
    C. Specific learning disorder is equally common among males and females.
    D. Prevalence rates vary according to the range of ages in the sample, selection criteria, severity of specific learning disorder, and academic domains investigated.
    E. Gender ratios cannot be attributed to factors such as ascertainment bias, definitional or measurement variation, language, race, or socioeconomic status.

**Correct Answer: C. Specific learning disorder is equally common among males and females.**

**Explanation:** Specific learning disorder is more common in males than in females (ratios range from about 2:1 to 3:1 and cannot be attributed to factors such as ascertainment bias, definitional or measurement variation, language, race, or socioeconomic status). The prevalence of specific learning disorder across the academic domains of reading, writing, and mathematics is approximately 5%–15% among school-age children across different languages and cultures. Prevalence in adults is unknown but appears to be approximately 4%.

**48—Specific Learning Disorder / Prevalence (p. 70); Gender-Related Diagnostic Issues (p. 73)**

49. Which of the following statements about comorbidity in specific learning disorder is *true?*

    A. Attention-deficit/hyperactivity disorder (ADHD) does not co-occur with specific learning disorder more frequently than would be expected by chance.
    B. Speech sound disorder and specific language impairments are not commonly comorbid with specific learning disorder.
    C. Identified clusters of co-occurrences include severe reading disorders; fine motor problems and handwriting problems; and problems with arithmetic, reading, and gross motor planning.
    D. The co-occurrence of specific learning disorder and specific language impairments has been shown in up to 20% of children with language problems.
    E. Co-occurring disorders generally do not influence the course or treatment of specific learning disorder.

    **Correct Answer: C. Identified clusters of co-occurrences include severe reading disorders; fine motor problems and handwriting problems; and problems with arithmetic, reading, and gross motor planning.**

    **Explanation:** Specific learning disorder commonly co-occurs with neurodevelopmental (e.g., ADHD, communication disorders, developmental coordination disorder, autistic spectrum disorder) or other mental disorders (e.g., anxiety disorders, depressive and bipolar disorders). These comorbidities do not necessarily exclude the diagnosis of specific learning disorder but may make testing and differential diagnosis more difficult, because each of the co-occurring disorders independently interferes with the execution of activities of daily living, including learning. Thus, clinical judgment is required to attribute such impairment to learning difficulties. If there is an indication that another diagnosis could account for the difficulties learning keystone academic skills described in Criterion A, specific learning disorder should not be diagnosed. Co-occurring disorders generally do influence the course or treatment, and when a child/adolescent is being evaluated, co-occurring disorders should be listed.

    **49—Specific Learning Disorder / Comorbidity (p. 74)**

50. Which of the following statements about developmental coordination disorder (DCD) is *true?*

    A. Some children with DCD show additional (usually suppressed) motor activity, such as choreiform movements of unsupported limbs or mirror movements.
    B. The prevalence of DCD in children ages 5–11 years is 1%–3%.
    C. In early adulthood, there is improvement in learning new tasks involving complex/automatic motor skills, including driving and using tools.

D. DCD has no association with prenatal exposure to alcohol or with low birth weight or preterm birth.

E. Impairments in underlying neurodevelopmental processes have not been found to primarily affect visuomotor skills.

**Correct Answer: A. Some children with DCD show additional (usually suppressed) motor activity, such as choreiform movements of unsupported limbs or mirror movements.**

**Explanation:** In regard to the choreiform or mirror movements seen in DCD, DSM-5 states, "these 'overflow' movements are referred to as *neurodevelopmental immaturities* or *neurological soft signs* rather than neurological abnormalities. In both current literature and clinical practice, their role in diagnosis is still unclear, requiring further evaluation." The prevalence of DCD in children ages 5–11 years is 5%–6% (in children age 7 years, 1.8% are diagnosed with severe DCD and 3% with probable DCD). In adulthood, there are often ongoing problems with learning new tasks involving complex/automatic motor skills. DCD is more common following prenatal exposure to alcohol and in preterm and low-birth-weight children. In DCD, deficits have been identified in both visuomotor perception and spatial mentalizing; these deficits affect the ability to make rapid motoric adjustments as the complexity of the required movements increases.

**50—Developmental Coordination Disorder / Associated Features Supporting Diagnosis; Prevalence; Risk and Prognostic Factors (pp. 75, 76)**

51. Which of the following statements about developmental coordination disorder (DCD) is *true?*

A. The disorder is usually not diagnosed before the age of 7 years.
B. Symptoms have usually improved significantly at 1-year follow-up.
C. In most cases, symptoms are no longer evident by adolescence.
D. DCD has no clear relationship with prenatal alcohol exposure, preterm birth, or low birth weight.
E. Cerebellar dysfunction is hypothesized to play a role in DCD.

**Correct Answer: E. Cerebellar dysfunction is hypothesized to play a role in DCD.**

**Explanation:** DCD is usually not diagnosed before 5 years of age, and the course has been demonstrated to be stable up to 1-year follow-up. In about 50%–70% of cases, symptoms continue into adolescence. Prenatal alcohol exposure, prematurity, and low birth weight may be risk factors.

**51—Developmental Coordination Disorder / Development and Course (p. 75)**

52. Which of the following is *not* a criterion for the DSM-5 diagnosis of stereotypic movement disorder?

    A. Motor behaviors are present that are repetitive, seemingly driven, and apparently purposeless.
    B. Onset of the behaviors is in the early developmental period.
    C. The behaviors result in self-inflicted bodily injury that requires medical treatment.
    D. The behaviors are not attributable to the physiological effects of a substance or neurological condition or better explained by another neurodevelopmental or mental disorder.
    E. The behaviors interfere with social, academic, or other activities.

    **Correct Answer: C. The behaviors result in self-inflicted bodily injury that requires medical treatment.**

    **Explanation:** Although the repetitive behaviors *may* result in self-injury, that is not a criterion for the diagnosis. All of the other options represent criteria for the diagnosis of stereotypic movement disorder.

    **52—Stereotypic Movement Disorder / diagnostic criteria (p. 77)**

53. Which of the following statements about the developmental course of stereotypic movement disorder is *false?*

    A. The presence of stereotypic movements may indicate an undetected neurodevelopmental problem, especially in children ages 1–3 years.
    B. Among typically developing children, the repetitive movements may be stopped when attention is directed to them or when the child is distracted from performing them.
    C. In some children, the stereotypic movements would result in self-injury if protective measures were not used.
    D. Whereas simple stereotypic movements (e.g., rocking) are common in young typically developing children, complex stereotypic movements are much less common (approximately 3%–4%).
    E. Stereotypic movements typically begin within the first year of life.

    **Correct Answer: E. Stereotypic movements typically begin within the first year of life.**

    **Explanation:** The movements typically begin within the first 3 years of life. Simple stereotypic movements are common in infancy and may be involved in acquisition of motor mastery. In children who develop complex motor stereotypies, approximately 80% exhibit symptoms before 24 months of age, 12% between 24 and 35 months, and 8% at 36 months or older.

    **53—Stereotypic Movement Disorder / Development and Course (p. 79)**

54. Which of the following is a DSM-5 diagnostic criterion for Tourette's disorder?

   A. Tics occur throughout a period of more than 1 year, and during this period there was never a tic-free period of more than 3 consecutive months.
   B. Onset is before age 5 years.
   C. The tics may wax and wane in frequency but have persisted for more than 1 year since first tic onset.
   D. Motor tics must precede vocal tics.
   E. The tics may occur many times a day for at least 4 weeks, but no longer than 12 consecutive months.

   **Correct Answer: C. The tics may wax and wane in frequency but have persisted for more than 1 year since first tic onset.**

   **Explanation:** Only option C is a criterion for the DSM-5 diagnosis of Tourette's disorder. In DSM-IV, Criterion B specified that tics must have been present for "a period of more than 1 year, and during this period there was never a tic-free period of more than 3 consecutive months." In DSM-5 this criterion was simplified to the requirement that tics must have persisted for more than 1 year since first tic onset.

   **54—Tic Disorders / diagnostic criteria (p. 81)**

55. At her child's third office visit, the mother of an 8-year-old boy with a 6-month history of excessive eye blinking and intermittent chirping says that she has noticed the development of grunting sounds since he started school this term. What is the most likely diagnosis?

   A. Tourette's disorder.
   B. Provisional tic disorder.
   C. Temporary tic disorder.
   D. Persistent (chronic) vocal tic disorder.
   E. Transient tic disorder, recurrent.

   **Correct Answer: B. Provisional tic disorder.**

   **Explanation:** The presence of single or multiple motor and/or vocal tics for *less* than 1 year meets Criteria A and B for provisional tic disorder. This is in contrast to Tourette's disorder, where tics must be present for *more* than 1 year. Thus, option A is incorrect. There is no such disorder as temporary tic disorder (option C). Persistent (chronic) vocal tic disorder (option D) is incorrect because in this vignette the boy has *both* motor and vocal tics, and they have been present for less than 1 year. Transient tic disorder, recurrent (option E), would have been correct if the question were asking for a DSM-IV diagnosis; however, transient tic disorder has been revised and renamed provisional tic disorder in DSM-5.

   **55—Tic Disorders / diagnostic criteria (p. 81)**

56. A 5-year-old girl is referred to your care with a DSM-IV diagnosis of chronic motor or vocal tic disorder. Under DSM-5, she would meet criteria for persistent (chronic) motor or vocal tic disorder. Which of the following statements about her new diagnosis under DSM-5 is *false?*

    A. She may have single or multiple motor or vocal tics, but not both.
    B. Her tics must persist for more than 1 year since first tic onset without a tic-free period for 3 consecutive months to meet diagnostic criteria.
    C. Her tics may wax and wane in frequency but have persisted for more than 1 year since first tic onset.
    D. She has never met criteria for Tourette's disorder.
    E. A specifier may be added to the diagnosis of persistent (chronic) motor or vocal tic disorder to indicate whether the girl has motor or vocal tics.

    **Correct Answer: B. Her tics must persist for more than 1 year since first tic onset without a tic-free period for 3 consecutive months to meet diagnostic criteria.**

    **Explanation:** Under DSM-5 criteria for persistent (chronic) motor or vocal tic disorder, tics may wax and wane. There is also no longer a requirement for a tic-free period. Thus, option C is true, and option B is the false statement. Options A and D are diagnostic criteria that are true for this classification under both DSM-IV and DSM-5. Option E is true because in DSM-5, one can specify "motor tics only" or "vocal tics only."

    **56—Tic Disorders / diagnostic criteria (p. 81)**

57. A highly functional 20-year-old college student with a history of anxiety symptoms and attention-deficit/hyperactivity disorder, for which she is prescribed lisdexamfetamine (Vyvanse), tells her psychiatrist that she has been researching the side effects of her medication for one of her class projects. In addition, she says that for the past week she has been feeling stressed by her schoolwork, and her friends have been asking her why she intermittently bobs her head up and down multiple times a day. What is the most likely diagnosis?

    A. Provisional tic disorder.
    B. Unspecified tic disorder.
    C. Unspecified anxiety disorder.
    D. Obsessive-compulsive personality disorder.
    E. Unspecified stimulant-induced disorder.

    **Correct Answer: B. Unspecified tic disorder.**

    **Explanation:** Given the data provided by the vignette, unspecified tic disorder (option B) is the best answer. Included in this category are presentations in which there is uncertainty about whether the tic is attributable to medication versus primary. By definition, onset must be before age 18 years for all tic disorders. Tic onset after 18 years of age would be diagnosed as unspecified tic disorder. Option E is incorrect given that the student is highly functioning, lacks significant impairment in her life (based on the limited details provided in the vignette), and takes lisdexamfetamine (Vyvanse), which may have less abuse potential since it is a prodrug.

**57—Tic Disorders / Differential Diagnosis (p. 84)**

58. Which of the following is *not* a DSM-5 diagnostic criterion for language disorder?

A. Persistent difficulties in the acquisition and use of language across modalities due to deficits in comprehension or production.
B. Language abilities that are substantially and quantifiably below those expected for age.
C. Symptom onset in the early developmental period.
D. Inability to attribute difficulties to hearing or other sensory impairment, motor dysfunction, or another medical or neurological condition.
E. Failure to meet criteria for mixed receptive-expressive language disorder or a pervasive developmental disorder.

**Correct Answer: E. Failure to meet criteria for mixed receptive-expressive language disorder or a pervasive developmental disorder.**

**Explanation:** Options A through D constitute the DSM-5 diagnostic criteria for language disorder. This diagnosis replaced the DSM-IV diagnoses expressive language disorder and mixed receptive-expressive language disorder. Option E is a criterion for expressive language disorder in DSM-IV and is thus incorrect. In contrast to DSM-IV, in DSM-5 meeting criteria for pervasive developmental disorder does not preclude one from being diagnosed with language disorder.

**58—Language Disorder / diagnostic criteria (p. 42)**

59. Which of the following statements about speech sound disorder is *true?*

A. Speech sound production must be present by age 2 years.
B. "Failure to use developmentally expected speech sounds" is assessed by comparison of a child with his or her peers of the same age and dialect.
C. The difficulties in speech sound production need not result in functional impairment to meet diagnostic criteria.
D. Symptom onset is in the early developmental period.
E. Both A and C are true.

**Correct Answer: D. Symptom onset is in the early developmental period.**

**Explanation:** The diagnosis of speech sound disorder in DSM-5 replaces the diagnosis of phonological disorder in DSM-IV. According to DSM-IV, Criterion A in the classification of phonological disorder is the "failure to use developmentally expected speech sounds that are appropriate for age and dialect." This has been revised in DSM-5 such that presence of "persistent difficulties in speech sound production that interfere with communication" suffices for Criterion A. Thus, option B is incorrect. There is also no specific age at onset for symptoms in speech sound disorder, but Criterion C specifies that symptom onset must be in the early developmental period. Thus, options A and E are incorrect, and D is the correct answer. Option C is a false statement, because Criterion B of speech sound disorder *does* require that difficulties from speech sound production interfere with one's function in social, academic, and occupational performance.

**59—Speech Sound Disorder / diagnostic criteria (p. 44)**

60. A mother brings her 4-year-old son to you for an evaluation with concerns that her son has struggled with speech articulation since very young. He has not sustained any head injuries, is otherwise healthy, and has a normal IQ. His preschool teacher reports that she does not always understand what he is saying and that other children tease him by calling him a "baby" due to his difficulty with communication. He does not have trouble relating to other people or understanding nonverbal social cues. What is the most likely diagnosis?

    A. Selective mutism.
    B. Global developmental delay.
    C. Speech sound disorder.
    D. Avoidant personality disorder.
    E. Unspecified anxiety disorder.

**Correct Answer: C. Speech sound disorder.**

**Explanation:** In this vignette, the child exhibits "persistent difficulty with speech sound production that interferes with speech intelligibility" leading to functional limitations in effective communication that interfere with social participation. Additionally, his symptoms are not attributable to a congenital or acquired medical condition and his symptom onset is in the early developmental period. These are the criteria for speech sound disorder. Option A is incorrect because the boy's difficulty in communication is in the sound production, rather than lack of communication during specific situations. Children who are selectively mute do not have difficulty with speech production. Option B is also incorrect because apart from difficulty with speech sound production, the boy relates well to other people and understands nonverbal cues. Option D is incorrect because the boy is too young to be diagnosed with an avoidant personality disorder; patterns of such behavior would be evident in early adulthood. Finally, although the boy may have some anxiety symptoms, this is difficult to assess without additional information. Thus, option E is incorrect.

**60—Speech Sound Disorder / diagnostic criteria (p. 44)**

61. A 6-year-old boy is failing school and continues to struggle significantly with grammar, sentence construction, and vocabulary. When he speaks, he also interjects "and" in between all his words. His teacher reports that he requires more verbal redirection than other students in order to stay on task. He is generally quiet and does not cause trouble otherwise. Which of the following diagnoses would be on your differential?

A. Language disorder.
B. Expressive language disorder.
C. Childhood-onset fluency disorder.
D. Attention-deficit/hyperactivity disorder (ADHD).
E. A and D.

**Correct Answer: E. Language disorder and ADHD.**

**Explanation:** This question asks for DSM-5 *diagnoses,* so option B is incorrect because expressive and mixed receptive-expressive language disorders are from DSM-IV. They are now consolidated into *language disorder* in DSM-5. Option A, language disorder, would be an important consideration in the differential diagnosis because the boy has persistent difficulties with both the production and possibly comprehension of language. The boy may need additional repetition to understand commands and may not interact with peers as readily due to communication difficulty, and thus appears quiet. Option C is incorrect because word interjections (e.g., "and") are no longer considered a type of speech disturbance in DSM-5. ADHD is a potential consideration given this boy's difficulty in staying on task and his poor academic performance. Thus, option E is the correct answer, and both language disorder and ADHD are diagnostic possibilities.

**61—Language Disorder / Comorbidity (p. 44)**

62. Which of the following types of disturbance in normal speech fluency/time patterning included in the DSM-IV criteria for stuttering was omitted in the DSM-5 criteria for childhood-onset fluency disorder (stuttering)?

A. Sound prolongation.
B. Circumlocution.
C. Interjections.
D. Words produced with an excess of physical tension.
E. Sound and syllable repetitions.

**Correct Answer: C. Interjections.**

**Explanation:** Criterion A for childhood-onset fluency disorder in DSM-5 requires the presence of one or more of seven types of disturbances, including those listed in options A, B, D, and E. The other speech fluency disturbances are broken words, audible or silent blocking, and monosyllabic whole-word repetitions. "Interjections" (option C) is the only fluency disturbance for stuttering in the DSM-IV criteria that was omitted in the DSM-5 criteria.

**62—Childhood-Onset Fluency Disorder (Stuttering) / diagnostic criteria (p. 45)**

63. A 14-year-old boy in regular education tells you that he thinks a girl in class likes him. His mother is surprised to hear this, because she reports that, since a young age, he has often struggled with making inferences or understanding nuances from what other people say. The teacher has also noticed that he sometimes misses nonverbal cues. He tends to get along better with adults, perhaps because they are not as likely to be put off by his overly formal speech. When he makes jokes, his peers do not always find the humor appropriate. Although he enjoys spending time with his best friend, he can be talkative and struggles with taking turns in conversation. What is the most likely diagnosis?

 A. Social (pragmatic) communication disorder.
 B. Asperger's disorder.
 C. Autism spectrum disorder.
 D. Social anxiety disorder.
 E. Language disorder.

**Correct Answer: A. Social (pragmatic) communication disorder.**

**Explanation:** Social (pragmatic) communication disorder is a new DSM-5 diagnosis characterized by "persistent difficulties in the social use of verbal and nonverbal communication as manifested by all of the following: 1) deficits in using communication for social purposes…in a manner that is appropriate for the social context, 2) impairment in the ability to change communication to match context or needs of the listener, 3) difficulties following rules for conversation and storytelling…and knowing how to use verbal and nonverbal signals to regulate interaction, [and] 4) difficulties understanding what is not explicitly stated." These deficits present in the early development period and result in functional limitations. Options B and C are incorrect because, respectively, Asperger's disorder is no longer a classification in DSM-5, and if this boy had autism he would likely be more impaired and unable to sustain a conversation. Option D is incorrect because social anxiety disorder would not affect one's ability to understand nuances in verbal and nonverbal communication. Option E is incorrect because the boy does not have difficulty with the production or comprehension of language, but rather with the nuances and social appropriateness of language content.

**63—Social (Pragmatic) Communication Disorder / Differential Diagnosis (p. 49)**

64. A 15-year-old boy with a prior diagnosis of Tourette's disorder is referred to your care. His mother tells you that during middle school he was teased for having vocal and motor tics. Since starting ninth grade, his tics have become less frequent. Currently, only mild motor tics remain. What is the appropriate DSM-5 diagnosis?

A. Tourette's disorder.
B. Persistent (chronic) motor tic disorder.
C. Provisional tic disorder.
D. Unspecified tic disorder.
E. Persistent (chronic) vocal tic disorder.

**Correct Answer: A. Tourette's disorder.**

**Explanation:** There are four tic disorder diagnostic categories, and they follow a hierarchical order: 1) Tourette's disorder, 2) persistent (chronic) motor or vocal tic disorder, 3) provisional tic disorder, and 4) unspecified tic disorder. According to Criterion E for tic disorders in DSM-5, once someone is diagnosed with a tic disorder at one level of the hierarchy, a diagnosis that is lower in the hierarchy cannot be made. In this case, option A is the correct answer because the boy has already been previously diagnosed with Tourette's disorder, which is at the top of the tic disorder hierarchy. Thus, at this point, he can no longer be diagnosed with persistent (chronic) motor tic disorder (option B). Options C and D are incorrect.

**64—Tic Disorders / diagnostic criteria (p. 81)**

65. Tics typically present for the first time during which developmental stage?

A. Infancy.
B. Prepuberty.
C. Latency.
D. Adolescence.
E. Adulthood.

**Correct Answer: B. Prepuberty.**

**Explanation:** Although it is not uncommon for adolescents and adults to present for an initial diagnostic assessment for tics, the initial onset of tics generally occurs during the prepubertal stage (ages 4–6 years). Tics then reach peak severity around ages 10–12 years, followed by a decline during adolescence. The incidence of new tic disorders decreases during the teen years, and even more so during adulthood. Clinicians should be wary of new-onset abnormal movements suggestive of tics outside of the usual age range.

**65—Tic Disorders / Development and Course (p. 83)**

66. A 7-year-old boy who has speech delays presents with long-standing, repetitive hand waving, arm flapping, and finger wiggling. His mother reports that she first noticed these symptoms when he was a toddler and wonders whether they are tics. She says that he tends to flap more when he is engrossed in activities, such as while watching his favorite television program, but will stop when called or distracted. Based on the mother's report, which of the following conditions would be highest on your list of possible diagnoses?

A. Provisional tic disorder.
B. Persistent (chronic) motor or vocal tic disorder.
C. Chorea.
D. Dystonia.
E. Motor stereotypies.

**Correct Answer: E. Motor stereotypies.**

**Explanation:** The boy's movements are not tics, but stereotypies. *Motor stereotypies* are defined as involuntary rhythmic, repetitive, predictable movements that appear purposeful but serve no obvious adaptive function or purpose and stop with distraction. Motor stereotypies can be differentiated from tics based on the former's earlier age at onset (younger than 3 years), prolonged duration (seconds to minutes), constant repetitive fixed form and location, exacerbation when engrossed in activities, lack of a premonitory urge, and cessation with distraction (e.g., name called or touched). Clinical history is crucial for differentiation.

*Chorea* represents rapid, random, continual, abrupt, irregular, unpredictable, nonstereotyped actions that are usually bilateral and affect all parts of the body (i.e., face, trunk, and limbs). The timing, direction, and distribution of movements vary from moment to moment, and movements usually worsen during attempted voluntary action. *Dystonia* is the simultaneous sustained contracture of both agonist and antagonist muscles, resulting in a distorted posture or movement of parts of the body. Dystonic postures are often triggered by attempts at voluntary movements and are not seen during sleep. The boy's movements do not fit these categories.

**66—Stereotypic Movement Disorder / Differential Diagnosis (p. 84)**

67. Assessment of co-occurring conditions is important for understanding the overall functional consequence of tics on an individual. Which of the following conditions has been associated with tic disorders?

    A. Attention-deficit/hyperactivity disorder (ADHD).
    B. Obsessive-compulsive and related disorders.
    C. Other movement disorders.
    D. Depressive disorders.
    E. All of the above.

**Correct Answer: E. All of the above.**

**Explanation:** Many medical and psychiatric conditions have been described as co-occurring with tic disorders, with ADHD and obsessive-compulsive and related disorders being particularly common. Children with ADHD may demonstrate disruptive behavior, social immaturity, and learning difficulties that may interfere with academic progress and interpersonal relationships and lead to greater impairment than that caused by a tic disorder. Individuals with tic disorders can also have other movement disorders and other mental disorders, such as depressive, bipolar, or substance use disorders.

**67—Tic Disorders / Comorbidity (p. 85)**

68. By what age should most children have acquired adequate speech and language ability to understand and follow social rules of verbal and nonverbal communication, follow rules for conversation and storytelling, and change language according to the needs of the listener or situation?

    A. Ages 2–3 years.
    B. Ages 3–4 years.
    C. Ages 4–5 years.
    D. Ages 5–6 years.
    E. Ages 6–7 years.

**Correct Answer: C. Ages 4–5 years.**

**Explanation:** Because social (pragmatic) communication depends on adequate developmental progress in speech and language, diagnosis of social (pragmatic) communication disorder is rare among children younger than 4 years. By age 4 or 5 years, most children should possess adequate speech and language abilities to permit identification of specific deficits in social communication. Milder forms of the disorder may not become apparent until early adolescence, when language and social interactions become more complex.

**68—Social (Pragmatic) Communication Disorder / Development and Course (p. 48)**

69. Having a family history of which of the following psychiatric disorders increases an individual's risk of social (pragmatic) communication disorder?

    A. Social anxiety disorder (social phobia).
    B. Autism spectrum disorder.
    C. Attention-deficit/hyperactivity disorder (ADHD).
    D. Specific learning disorder.
    E. Either B or D.

**Correct Answer: E. Either B or D.**

**Explanation:** A family history of autism spectrum disorder, communication disorders, or specific learning disorder appears to increase the risk of social (pragmatic) communication disorder. Although deficits stemming from ADHD and social anxiety disorder (social phobia) may overlap with symptoms of social communication disorder and may represent important considerations in the differential diagnosis, their presence in an individual's family history is not currently known to increase that person's risk of social (pragmatic) communication disorder.

**69—Social (Pragmatic) Communication Disorder / Development and Course (p. 48)**

70. A 6-year-old boy with a history of mild language delay is brought to your office by his mother, who is concerned that he is being teased in school because he misinterprets nonverbal cues and speaks in overly formal language with his peers. She tells you that her son was in an early intervention program, but his written and spoken language is now at grade level. The boy does not have a history of repetitive movements, sensory issues, or ritualized behaviors. Although he prefers constancy, he adapts fairly well to new situations. Additionally, he has a long-standing interest in trains and cars and is able to recite for you all the car models he memorized from a book on the history of transportation. Which of the following disorders would be a primary consideration in the differential diagnosis?

    A. Social (pragmatic) communication disorder.
    B. Autism spectrum disorder.
    C. Global developmental delay.
    D. Language disorder.
    E. A and B.

    **Correct Answer: A. Social (pragmatic) communication disorder.**

    **Explanation:** The presence of restricted interests and repetitive behaviors, interests, and activities beginning from early development is the primary diagnostic difference between autism spectrum disorder and social (pragmatic) communication disorder. In this vignette, the boy does not meet Criterion B for autism spectrum disorder, which requires evidence of at least two restricted, repetitive patterns of behavior, interests, or activities. Furthermore, although the boy has an interest in cars and trains, these are not necessarily atypical interests for boys at his age. Option E is also incorrect because in addition to the aforementioned reason, the two diagnoses are mutually exclusive. According to DSM-5, an individual who shows impairment in social communication and social interactions but does not show restricted and repetitive behavior or interests may meet criteria for social communication disorder instead of autism spectrum disorder. "The diagnosis of autism spectrum disorder supersedes that of social (pragmatic) communication disorder whenever the criteria for autism spectrum disorder are met, and care should be taken to enquire carefully regarding past or current restricted/repetitive behavior." Option D is incorrect because, from the limited data in the case, the mother suggests that his language is no longer a problem. Similarly, although option C would also be a consideration in the differential diagnosis, it is not the best answer given the data.

    **70—Social (Pragmatic) Communication Disorder / Differential Diagnosis (p. 49)**

71. Below what age is it difficult to distinguish a language disorder from normal developmental variations?

    A. Age 2 years.
    B. Age 3 years.

C. Age 4 years.
D. Age 5 years.
E. Age 6 years.

**Correct Answer: C. Age 4 years.**

**Explanation:** During the early developmental period, there is significant variation in early language acquisition, and it may be difficult to distinguish normal variations from impairments. By the time a child is 4 years old, language ability becomes more stable.

**71—Language Disorder / Differential Diagnosis (p. 43)**

72. Which of the following psychiatric diagnoses is strongly associated with language disorder?

A. Attention-deficit/hyperactivity disorder.
B. Developmental coordination disorder.
C. Autism spectrum disorder.
D. Social (pragmatic) communication disorder.
E. All of the above.

**Correct Answer: E. All of the above.**

**Explanation:** Language disorder is strongly associated with other neurodevelopmental disorders in terms of specific learning disorder (literacy and numeracy), attention-deficit/hyperactivity disorder, autism spectrum disorder, and developmental coordination disorder. It is also associated with social (pragmatic) communication disorder. A positive family history of speech or language disorders is often present.

**72—Language Disorder / Comorbidity (p. 44)**

73. Which of the following statements about the development of speech as it applies to speech sound disorder is *false?*

A. Most children with speech sound disorder respond well to treatment.
B. Speech sound production should be mostly intelligible by age 3 years.
C. Most speech sounds should be pronounced clearly and accurately according to age and community norms before age 10 years.
D. Lisping may or may not be associated with speech sound disorder.
E. It is abnormal for children to shorten words when they are learning to talk.

**Correct Answer: E. It is abnormal for children to shorten words when they are learning to talk.**

**Explanation:** Speech sound production requires both phonological knowledge and the ability to coordinate movements of the jaw, tongue, lips, and breath. A speech sound disorder is diagnosed when the speech sound production is not what is expected based on the child's age and developmental stage. Developmentally, children often shorten words and syllables when they are learning to talk, but by age 3–4 years, most of their speech should be intelligible. By age 7, most speech sounds should be articulated clearly according to age and community norms. Lisping is common in speech sound disorder and may be associated with an abnormal tongue-thrust swallowing pattern.

**73—Speech Sound Disorder (pp. 44–45)**

74. Which of the following would likely *not* be an important condition to rule out in the differential diagnosis of speech sound disorder?

   A. Normal variations in speech.
   B. Hearing or other sensory impairment.
   C. Dysarthria.
   D. Depression.
   E. Selective mutism.

**Correct Answer: D. Depression.**

**Explanation:** All of the options except option D are important considerations when making a diagnosis of speech sound disorder. Regional and cultural variations are important to consider, as well as abnormalities of speech due to hearing impairments. Dysarthria includes speech impairments due to a motor disorder and must also be considered, especially since this may be difficult to differentiate in young children. Selective mutism may be due to embarrassment or shyness.

**74—Speech Sound Disorder / Differential Diagnosis (p. 45)**

75. Which of the following statements about the development of childhood-onset fluency disorder (stuttering) is *true?*

   A. Stuttering occurs by age 6 for 80%–90% of affected individuals.
   B. Stuttering always begin abruptly and is noticeable to everyone.
   C. Stress and anxiety do not exacerbate disfluency.
   D. Motor movements are not associated with this disorder.
   E. None of the above.

**Correct Answer: A. Stuttering occurs by age 6 for 80%–90% of affected individuals.**

**Explanation:** The key feature of childhood-onset fluency disorder is a disturbance in the normal fluency and time patterning of speech that is inappropriate for the individual's age. Age at onset ranges from 2 to 7 years and occurs by age 6 for 80%–90% of affected individuals. Disfluencies can be gradual or sudden, and even subtle (thus, option B is incorrect). Emotional stress or anxiety can exacerbate stuttering, and motor movements may sometimes accompany this disorder (thus, options C and D are incorrect).

**75—Childhood-Onset Fluency Disorder (Stuttering) (pp. 45–47)**